Hashimoto's Thyroiditis
Hypothyroidism
Fatigue

Questions from Real Patients

By

Shunzhong Shawn Bao, MD

Editor: Barbara Winter

Ace Health Publisher

Publisher's Note/Disclaimer

The information contained herein is not intended to replace the services of a trained health professional or to be a substitute for individual medical advice. You should consult with your healthcare professional regarding to any matter related to your health, and in particular, any matter that may require diagnosis and medical attention.

First Edition 2018

Hashimoto's Thyroiditis
Hypothyroidism
Fatigue

Questions from Real Patients
Not Just Pills
Shunzhong Shawn Bao, MD
Barbara Winter, Editor

Published by Ace Health Publisher

Dedication

This book is dedicated to my patients. These are their intelligent questions for which I am grateful. They motivate me to think, continue learning and improving my patient care every day. These days, doctors do not have enough time to address all the questions patients may have. I hope my patients will get some answers here.

I want to thank my nurses, Betty Westbury, Carla Stacks, Walter Chavis who are providing excellent care to my patients and were the first readers of this book. With their critiques, they have made significant contributions.

This book is also dedicated to my good friend, my editor, Barbara Winter, for her unending kindness and generosity. With her patience and critical editing, she has made this book readable.

Finally, this book is dedicated to my wife who deserves deep, enduring gratitude, and also to my two children who are both in medical school. They are "first round editors". They helped me despite their heavy medical school work. They inspire me to learn and strive for excellence in patient care.

Preface

Hashimoto's thyroiditis is a relatively common condition. When people hear this diagnosis their first reaction is "what is that?" In this book I answer questions like this one and also questions about possible causes and available treatment. In addition, I address questions about diet and its relationship to Hashimoto's thyroiditis.

I want to help you thoroughly understand this disease. I have a patient who was diagnosed with Hashimoto's thyroiditis. She tried to cure it with some diet. She soon developed myxedema which is the most severe kind of hypothyroidism and nearly died. In what follows I want to help you truly understand the root cause of Hashimoto's thyroiditis and its evidence-based medical treatment thus avoiding the mistake this woman made.

This book is not just to help you understand Hashimoto's thyroiditis, but to also help you understand fatigue which is one of the most common and most distressful conditions people associate with the disease. I described 13 cases of Hashimoto's thyroiditis and fatigue. Each case is presented in detail. Patients, as well as young doctors, can learn from these cases.

While providing very practical guidelines for patients, this book addresses specific questions such as how to prepare for some common thyroid tests, how to take thyroid medications, etc.

Patients with Hashimoto's thyroiditis, or who have a family history of thyroid conditions, as well as those who just want to learn more about the disease will all benefit from reading this book and keeping it as a reference.

Contents

Chapter 1. The Basics of Thyroid and Diagnosis of Hashimoto's Thyroiditis

What is thyroid?

In English "thyroid gland" is derived from the Latin Glandula Thyreoidea meaning "shield-shaped gland". It is located at the base of your neck.

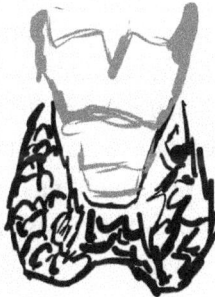

Fig. Illustration of thyroid gland at the base of neck.

The thyroid hormones are T3 and T4. T3 is the active hormone that affects every cell, every tissue, or organ in our body. It is crucial for cells to function properly.

What is Hashimoto's thyroiditis?

The name Hashimoto's thyroiditis came from the 1912 pathology paper by a Japanese doctor Hakaru Hashimoto. He described patients with goiter (big thyroid) and intense lymphocytic infiltration of the thyroid as "struma lymphomatosa". Later the paper was translated into English and in honor of him, we named the lymphocytic thyroiditis as Hashimoto's thyroiditis. This name has pathologic features, but we usually do not make the diagnosis based on the pathology.

Some doctors reserve this term only for patients with hypothyroidism (underactive thyroid). However, I make the diagnosis of Hashimoto's thyroiditis regardless of the thyroid's size and function.

How do you make the diagnosis of Hashimoto's thyroiditis?

I make the diagnosis of Hashimoto's diagnosis based on thyroid autoantibodies. If any antibody common commercially available tests is positive, then I give my patients the diagnosis of Hashimoto's thyroiditis. The thyroid can be enlarged, small or normal. If there is concurrent abnormal thyroid functioning, the diagnosis is confirmed. If their thyroid function is absolutely normal, and the patient does not have any symptoms, I might proceed with thyroid ultrasound. If the ultrasound does not show any sign of Hashimoto's thyroiditis, the increased TPO could be false positive, or the disease is at a very early stage and we might not need to treat.

I also make the diagnosis of Hashimoto's thyroiditis based on a thyroid ultrasound if I see a typical presentation of Hashimoto's thyroid, even when none of the antibodies are positive. This can be very complicated. As we know, other conditions can also have similar ultrasound features. Therefore, the diagnosis is not absolute. The good news is that if thyroid function is normal, we only need to follow, instead of treating.

I also made the diagnosis using Fine Needle Aspiration (FNA) for a few patients. This occurs most likely when the FNA was done for a nodule and the pathologist reported back as Hashimoto's thyroiditis.

Why do you add thyroid ultrasound results and Fine Needle Aspiration (FNA) as your diagnostic tools?

Thyroid peroxidase antibody (TPO) is very sensitive and can show a false positive. Also not all patients with Hashimoto's thyroiditis have positive TPO. Thyroid ultrasound is not super sensitive, but thyroid ultrasound can show typical changes.

Hashimoto's thyroiditis is inflammation of the thyroid which is caused by an autoimmune disease. The FNA can see some specific inflammation cells. I usually do not do FNA simply to make the diagnosis of Hashimoto's thyroiditis. We usually do FNA to make sure a nodule or nodular structure (lesion) is not cancerous. Although professional societies have not recommend to screen thyroid cancer in Hashimoto's thyroiditis, there are reports that revealed the thyroid cancer rate was 0.5-30% in patients with Hashimoto's thyroiditis.

Why do you only test TPO?

Someone did a study and found that in a group of patients of both positive TPO and antithyroglobulin antibodies, only 1% of patients positive for antithyroglobulin were negative for TPO.

If the TPO is negative, but I still suspect the patient has Hashimoto's thyroiditis, I would then order antithyroglobulin antibody and do a thyroid ultrasound.

Is there any other antibody you test?

Sometimes, if the diagnosis is uncertain. I might order thyrotropin receptor antibody (TRab). Some specialists believe this antibody is more specific. The specificity and sensitivity of using this test in making the diagnosis is still not very reliable.

If your TSH is low or you have some symptoms of overactive thyroid. I will test thyroid stimulating immunoglobulin (TSI). TSI is also one of the TRab which stimulates your thyroid to grow (leads to goiter) and produce too much thyroid hormone. This test takes more time since it is a bioassay.

How many subtypes of Hashimoto's thyroiditis are there?

It was first classified into primary and secondary. Primary Hashimoto's thyroiditis is the most common. The exact cause is not very clear yet. We know it is the most common autoimmune disease and can also with other autoimmune diseases like rheumatoid arthritis, lupus, celiac disease, Type I Diabetes, and Sjogren's disease. Primary Hashimoto's thyroiditis can be subclassified into the following five types based on clinical presentations and pathological changes.

- Classic form: This is the most common, and the form Dr. Hashimoto described.
- Fibrous variant: This is a pathology term. There is marked presence of fibrous replacement of the thyroid parenchyma at the same time as significant lymphocytic replacement.
- IgG4 related variant: There is thyroid inflammation rich in IgG4-positive plasma cells and marked fibrosis. This variant is also diagnosed pathologically.
- Juvenile form: This is a clinical term. It simply means that Hashimoto's thyroiditis is diagnosed at childhood.

- Hashitoxicosis: Both features of Hashimoto's thyroiditis and Graves' disease (overactive thyroid) are present. I have two patients who were treated with levothyroxine for over 40 years and suddenly had overactive thyroid, so the Hashitoxicosis can occur sequentially also.
- Painless thyroiditis (sporadic and postpartum): This is also a clinical diagnosis.

What is secondary Hashimoto's thyroiditis?

Secondary Hashimoto's thyroiditis is caused by another disease or by medication. The most common reason is administration of immunomodulatory agents, like interferons for hepatitis C treatment or cancer immunotherapy. I also have patients whose secondary thyroiditis is caused by excessive iron deposits in the thyroid through hemochromatosis.

How do I know which type of Hashimoto's thyroiditis I have?

As we discussed that Hashimoto's thyroiditis is a combination of clinical and pathological diagnosis. Especially for fibrous variant and IgG4 variant are pathological diagnosis. Thyroid ultrasound can be helpful too.

The juvenile Hashimoto's thyroiditis, Hashitoxicosis and painless thyroiditis are more clinical diagnosis.

For secondary Hashimoto's thyroiditis is also clinical diagnosis. For patients who do not have thyroid condition before and then diagnosed Hashimoto's thyroiditis after immunotherapy.

What is the cause of primary Hashimoto's thyroiditis?

The exact cause is not clear yet. Scientists have been working on it since 1912. However, the disease has been recognized linked to the following:

- Your genes
  - Very often in the family. Doctors always ask your family history. The odds are very high that your mother, aunt or somebody else also has Hashimoto's thyroiditis.
  - Also very common in a family with Graves' disease (another autoimmune thyroid disease).
  - If your sister has Hashimoto's thyroiditis, your chance is increased 20-fold if you are also a female.
  - If your monozygotic twin has Hashimoto's thyroiditis, your chance to develop Hashimoto's thyroiditis is 30-60%.
  - Hashimoto's thyroiditis occurs with increased frequency in patients with Down syndrome and Turner syndrome.
- Virus infection
- Female gender. The female to male ratio is close to 1:10.
- Stress has been implicated in developing Hashimoto's thyroiditis.
- Pregnancy leads to lots of changes in our immune system. A condition called postpartum thyroiditis is a variant of Hashimoto's thyroiditis.
- Both iodine deficiency and excessive iodine are linked to increased risk for Hashimoto's thyroiditis.
- Radiation exposure or people who work in the field of medical radiation have higher risk. People exposed to nuclear power plant accidents also have increased risk.

I do not have goiter (large thyroid). Can I have Hashimoto's thyroiditis?

Hashimoto's thyroiditis can have normal thyroid size, smaller or larger thyroid. For most patients, during the disease process, the thyroid can become smaller and smaller.

My thyroid function is always normal. Can I have Hashimoto's thyroiditis?

Again, the diagnosis of Hashimoto's thyroiditis is not dependent on its function. It strictly depends on pathology. Clinically, most of the time, we make the diagnosis based on the lab tests of antibodies (see above). The thyroid function can be normal, low, high, or from low to high recycling.

What kind of symptoms can I have if I have Hashimoto's thyroiditis?

Most patients come to me for Hashimoto's thyroiditis because they think they have a thyroid condition already. Unfortunately, the symptoms are very non-specific. In other words, we cannot say because you have these symptoms you have Hashimoto's thyroiditis. One of the reasons is that the thyroid affects every cell, and every organ in our body. Therefore, abnormal thyroid can cause all different symptoms and signs. Patients like to attribute a lot of symptoms to their thyroid.

In case of Hashimoto's thyroiditis, it is more complicated than simple hypothyroidism like surgical hypothyroidism. Hashimoto's thyroiditis is the most common autoimmune disease and all autoimmune diseases tend to cluster. Some of the symptoms patients as well as doctors attribute to Hashimoto's thyroiditis could be caused by concurrent other autoimmune diseases. In the following few questions, we will discuss moderate to severe hypothyroidism.

What are the most common symptoms of Hashimoto's thyroiditis?

In my practice, the most common complaints are fatigue, not feeling well, and weight gain. Other less common symptoms are dry skin, dry hair, losing hair, brittle nails and foggy brain.

What is the manifestation in skin?

Moderate to severe hypothyroidism can cause the skin to be cool and pale. There are at least three reasons. One is that hypothyroidism causes decreased metabolism and your body produces less heat; The second reason is that your blood flow to the skin is reduced; The third reason is that you might have mild anemia. The epidermis has an atrophied cellular layer and hyperkeratosis that results in the characteristic dry roughness of the skin.

The following skin changes may also occur:

- Dry skin and coarse and roughness of the skin.
- Skin discoloration such as a yellowish tinge may be present if the patient has carotenemia. Since Hashimoto's thyroiditis can be clustered with other autoimmune diseases if the patient also has adrenal insufficiency (Addison's disease) increased darkness may be seen.
- Nonpitting edema (myxedema) occurs in severe hypothyroidism and may be generalized. It results from accumulation of the skin with something called glycosaminoglycans with associated water retention.

- Vitiligo and alopecia areata may be present, especially in patients with celiac disease and cycle between hypothyroidism and hyperthyroidism.
- Rash or skin light sensitivity may occur in patients with lupus.
- Raynaud's phenomenon: purple fingers and toes when cold.
- Idiopathic hives might be related to Hashimoto's thyroiditis.

What is the manifestation in the eyes?

Puffy eyes can occur if hypothyroidism is severe enough. Some patients also complain of heavy eyes. For patients who cycle between hyper and hypothyroidism they can have variations of staring and protrusion of the eyeballs.

What is the manifestation in the hematologic system?

Anemia is common. As we know, hypothyroidism slows down everything including the bone marrow system which is responsible for making blood cells.

Hashimoto's thyroiditis can concur with pernicious anemia. Pernicious anemia is also an autoimmune disease which destructs the stomach cells which produce something called intrinsic factor. Intrinsic factor is required for vitamin B12 absorption. Vitamin B12 is required for making DNA. I will talk more about pernicious anemia in this book since this is very important in managing Hashimoto's thyroiditis. 10% or more of Hashimoto's thyroiditis patients have pernicious anemia and they are not being diagnosed. This condition if not diagnosed has very severe consequences and if diagnosed, it is easy to treat.

Moderate to severe hypothyroidism can also cause iron deficiency which might be due to reduced iron absorption. In females at the reproductive age with menstrual periods, uncontrolled hypothyroidism leads to irregular, prolonged and heavy periods. Excessive blood loss can cause severe iron deficiency anemia.

What is the manifestation in the cardiovascular system?

Prolonged and moderate to severe hypothyroidism can cause heart failure. I reported a case of a 35-year-old female with undiagnosed severe hypothyroidism caused by Sheehan syndrome. Her severe hypothyroidism had not been diagnosed due to lack of insurance. When she was evaluated in the ER and the hospital for heart failure, just her TSH was checked. Her TSH was either normal or slightly off and the doctors thought it was due to a nonthyroidal illness. She lost her job and lost her husband and family. She was completely disabled. She was put on the heart transplant list. Her heart function was back to normal after nine months of thyroid treatment. If you want to learn more about this fascinating case, please google my name and read my publications.

Patients can have other conditions like pericardial effusion (too much fluid collecting around the heart).

Hypothyroidism that is not optimally treated can also increase the risk for coronary artery disease leading to heart attacks:
- Hypothyroidism reduces the metabolism. I have patients whose bad cholesterol was over 200 mg/dl and after being properly treated for hypothyroidism, the LDL came down below 100 mg/dl without cholesterol medication. Therefore, anyone who has high cholesterol should be screened for thyroid disease. I always start cholesterol medication after optimizing thyroid medication.

- Hypothyroidism causes hyperhomocysteinemia which is also a risk factor for coronary artery disease.
- Increased blood pressure-Hypothyroidism causes stiffness of blood vessels leading to uncontrolled hypertension.
- Unstable blood pressure-Hashimoto's thyroiditis can occur with other autoimmune conditions leading to dysautonomia (the autonomic nervous system regulates blood pressure).

All of these cause patients to have fatigue, lack of stamina, slow or fast heart rate, shortness of breath, or activity intolerance.

What is the manifestation in the respiratory system?

The respiratory system is closely linked to the cardiovascular system and causes similar symptoms like fatigue, shortness of breath, or physical activity intolerance.

Hypothyroidism can cause reduced lung capacity and oxygen and carbon dioxide exchange.

Hypothyroidism also is linked to obstructive sleep apnea and obesity. Both conditions can have severe consequences on the respiratory system.

Hypothyroidism is also believed to cause pulmonary hypertension which causes reduced lung capacity to perform its function and oxygen and carbon dioxide exchange.

Many interstitial lung diseases are autoimmune diseases. They can be presented together.

What is the manifestation in the digestive system?

Constipation is the most common complaint. This is most likely due to decreased gut motility. Small intestinal bacterial overgrowth may also contribute to gastrointestinal symptoms like bloating.

Other gastrointestinal problems that can occur in hypothyroidism are:

- Decreased taste sensation.
- Gastric atrophy due to the presence of antiparietal cell antibodies. Pernicious anemia occurs in 10 percent of patients with Hashimoto's thyroiditis.
- Celiac disease is four times more common in hypothyroid patients compared with the general population.
- Some of these conditions can cause severe nutritional deficiency.

What is the manifestation in the reproductive system?

Women with hypothyroidism may have menstruation problems: too little, too heavy, too long, too short, or amenorrhea. Fertility is reduced and the risk for abortion is significantly increased.

Hypothyroidism can cause increased prolactin (called hyperprolactinemia). Hyperprolactinemia may occur and is occasionally sufficiently severe enough to cause amenorrhea or galactorrhea (milk secretion without related to pregnancy).

Men with hypothyroidism may experience hypogonadism (low testosterone). This can cause low libido, erectile dysfunction, and delayed ejaculation. The sperm are also found to be abnormal.

- The serum sex hormone is reduced. If a mild case, sex binding globulin concentration may be low in hypothyroidism. This will lower serum total but not free sex hormone concentrations. In severe cases, free sex hormone can also be reduced. In these patients usually both their gonadotropins and testosterone levels are reduced.
- Hypothyroidism can cause obesity and obstructive sleep apnea which leads to low testosterone and also hypogonadism.

Autoimmune hypogonadism is an underdiagnosed condition. In men, there is no such description. In women, I have had patients with polyglandular disease. I will describe the case in a later chapter.

What is the manifestation in the nervous system?

Most common complaints patients have are brain fog and memory loss. A very severe case produces Hashimoto encephalopathy. Most severe cases can result in myxedema coma, while mild cases can be like carpal tunnel syndrome.

What is Hashimoto encephalopathy?

Severe cases described as Hashimoto encephalopathy are characterized as acute or subacute confusion with altered level of consciousness, seizures, and myoclonus (involuntary muscle jerks or twitches). The exact etiology is not clear. I consider this as autoimmune encephalitis. Encephalitis means "inflammation of the brain".

What is myxedema coma?

Myxedema coma is defined as the most severe hypothyroidism leading to decreased mental status, low body temperature, and other symptoms related to slowing of function in multiple organs. It is a medical emergency with a high mortality rate. Fortunately, it is now such a rare presentation of hypothyroidism, and I have never encountered one.

What is the manifestation in the musculoskeletal system?

Muscle involvement in adults with hypothyroidism is common. Patients may experience weakness, cramps, and myalgias (muscle pain). The serum creatine kinase (CK) is also frequently elevated. Joint pains, aches, and stiffness may also occur in patients with hypothyroidism. Gout has been reported more common in hypothyroid patients compared with the general population.

Chapter 2. Understanding Thyroid Function Tests

How is thyroid function regulated?

Lots of important hormones are regulated by the hypothalamus and pituitary gland. The pituitary gland is a central command for many hormones. It is situated at the base of the brain behind the nose. The hypothalamus secretes a hormone called the thyroid releasing hormone (TRH). It then promotes the pituitary gland to release another hormone called the thyroid stimulating hormone (TSH). TSH then stimulates the thyroid to synthesize and release thyroxine (T4) and triiodothyronine (T3). The levels of T3 and T4 regulate TSH by feedback.

What is TSH?

TSH is a hormone secreted from the pituitary gland. It works like a thermostat. If the T3 and T4 levels are too low, then the TSH levels are elevated. If the T3 and T4 levels are too high, then the TSH levels decline.

TSH regulates T4 and T3 release just like the thermostat regulates your house temperature. TSH is like the thermostat; T4, T3 are like the temperature at your house. If the temperature is too high, your thermostat will shut down; if the temperature is too low, your thermostat will start up. Therefore, if your T4 and T3 are too high, TSH will decrease; if T4 and T3 are too low, TSH will increase. Certainly, the assumption is that your thermostat works properly; likewise the assumption is that your pituitary works properly.

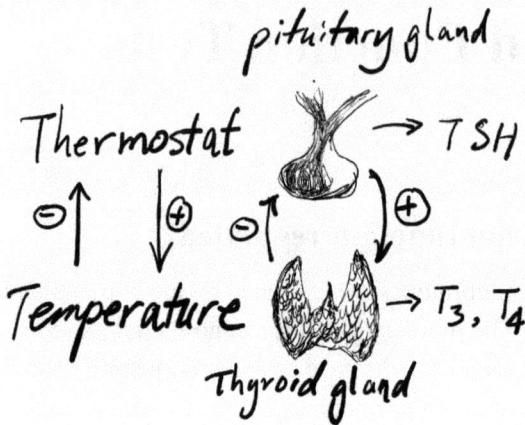

Fig. Illustration of the relationship between the pituitary hormone TSH and T3 and T4 just like a thermostat and the temperature. + indicating stimulating to cause T3 and T4 or temperature to increase; - indicating suppressing (feedback) to cause TSH to decrease or the thermostat to shut down, and then T3 and T4, and temperature to decrease.

What is the normal value for TSH?

Different labs might give different normal values. Most labs give a normal value of 0.5-5 mIU/L. At different ages, the normal value is slightly different. When we age the TSH value tends to increase slightly. At each stage in pregnancy the TSH levels are different.

What non-thyroid conditions and drugs might affect TSH levels?

Some specialists and professional societies only recommend checking TSH levels which can miss the full picture since your TSH can be affected by many conditions and medications. If you are very sick, your TSH can be low.

Lots of medications also affect TSH values. The most common medications are steroids, dopamine agonists (bromocriptine, cabergoline), somatostatin (a hormone from the pituitary gland or another gland to suppress other hormone secretion), amphetamine, metformin (diabetes medication), amiodarone (heart medication), rexinoids, and opioids.

Is it true that taking too high a dose of biotin can affect TSH measurement?

Yes, biotin might affect the laboratory measurement but not its function.

How are T3 and T4 measured?

Under normal conditions, our thyroid secretes 80% T4 and 20% T3. Most circulating T3 is converted from T4 to T3 in peripheral tissues like the liver or kidney. For T4, in blood, 99.98% is bound to proteins (thyroxine-binding globulin, transthyretin and albumin), while 99.80% of T3 is bound to proteins.

It is much easier and more accurate to measure the total hormone (protein bound+free). However, many conditions and medications can affect binding protein levels and then falsely affect the total hormone level. Therefore, I do not order the test of total hormone very often and the measurements for free hormones are not very accurate either.

17

What medications increase the total hormones but do not affect the thyroid's function?

- Estrogens
- Birth control pills
- Tamoxifen(for breast cancer)
- Mitotane
- Heroin
- 5-fluorouracil (5-FU, cancer medication)
- Methadone (addiction medication)

If you are told you have high thyroid hormone levels, you need to let your doctor know you are on these medications.

What medications decrease the total hormones but do not affect the thyroid's function?

Some medications can reduce the thyroid binding proteins and then the total hormone levels.

- Androgens (testosterone and similar hormones)
- Glucocorticoids (like prednisone)
- Lithium (can cause thyroid dysfunction)
- Phenytoin
- Propranolol (also inhibit the conversion from T4 to T3)
- Niacin (nicotinic acid)

What conditions increase thyroid hormone binding proteins and then increase the total hormones with normal thyroid function?

The following conditions might increase thyroid binding proteins and then increase the total hormone measurement:

- Pregnancy
- Acute /chronic liver disease (can go both ways)
- Adrenal insufficiency

- AIDS
- Familial dysalbuminemic hyperthyroxinemia is a type of hyperthyroxinemia associated with mutations in the human serum albumin gene.
- Familial hyperthyroxinemia due to increased thyroxine binding protein.

What conditions decrease thyroid binding proteins and then reduce the total thyroid hormones with normal thyroid function?

The following conditions might reduce the thyroid binding proteins and cause the measurement of total hormones to be decreased:

- Critical illness (very sick)
- Sepsis (blood infection)
- Nephrotic syndrome (lots of protein lost from kidneys). Recently I saw a person who actually developed hypothyroidism.
- Diabetic ketoacidosis (please read my diabetes book)
- Acute and chronic liver diseases (can go both ways)
- Chronic alcoholism
- Severe cirrhosis
- Severe malnutrition
- Acromegaly (enlarged body parts caused by a brain tumor secreting growth hormone)
- Cushing's syndrome or Cushing's disease (caused by an overabundance of steroids in the body)
- Familial thyroxine binding protein deficiency (gene mutation)

How do we measure Free T4 and Free T3?

The free unbound hormones are active; thus, it makes more sense to measure the free hormones. However, the measurement is not so accurate due to the very low level of the free hormones. Again, only 0.02% of T4 is free hormone and 0.2% of T3 is free hormone.

There are two ways to measure Free T4 and Free T3:
- Estimation of Free T4 and Free T3 testing.
    - o Use two assays to check both total T3, T4, and binding proteins and then calculate the index.
- Use automated immunoassay-most commonly clinically used.
    - o Direct measurement. It is very technically demanding and not routinely performed. In very special rare situations, I might order it.

What medication can affect automated immunoassay? I have an abnormal thyroid function test, but my function is normal.

Here are the common medications:
- Artificially increase Free T4
    - o Amiodarone (can truly increase T4 synthesis)
    - o Salicylate (greater than 2g/day)
    - o NSAIDS(nonsteroidal anti-inflammatory drugs)
    - o Biotin
    - o Heparin use
- Artificially decrease Free T4
    - o Seizure medication: phenytoin(dilantin)
    - o Seizure medication: carbamazepine

What is TPO?

TPO represents thyroperoxidase, but when we are talking about it most people are talking about the antibody of TPO. It is reported as a titer like 1: 120. When it is high, it usually means you have autoimmune thyroid disease-Hashimoto's thyroiditis.

Does TPO increase the risk of thyroid cancer?

It is reported that patients with autoimmune disease have higher risks for thyroid cancer. However, it is not concrete. Currently, no professional societies suggest that you have to screen for thyroid cancer if you have an autoimmune thyroid disease like Hashimoto's thyroiditis.

There is no concrete data suggesting that thyroid nodules in a patient with increased TPO antibody have a higher risk for cancer.

Why is my TPO up and down?

The unstable nature of autoimmune disease is the cause of TPO increasing or decreasing, but also remember the testing is not often accurate. The lab sometimes changes different assays which also confuses patients and doctors.

Therefore, please do not be too alarmed about TPO variations. I do not recommend checking them repeatedly.

Is there any treatment for increased TPO?

There is no concrete treatment. Some report that selenium might help. I recommend patients to take 100 mcg of selenium (or selenomethionine 200 mcg) daily. In some patients TPO decreases with the selenium supplement.

Can I take too much selenium?

Yes, you can have too much. We call it selenosis. We can check your blood level. If your blood level is over 100 mcg/dl, you have too much selenium. If you have too much selenium in your blood, you might develop nail problems, hair loss, skin rash, fatigue or increased irritability. Some also reported having garlic-smelling breath.

If more severe and long term, some cases of skin cancer, liver, or kidney damage are reported. I also saw reports that the overdose of selenium was linked to the development of diabetes.

What food do you recommend to increase my selenium level?

Healthy food like nuts and vegetables such as spinach have good levels of selenium.

What is thyroglobulin? Do I have higher thyroid cancer risks if my value is high?

Thyroglobulin is secreted from normal thyroid follicular cells. It correlates to thyroid volume. The bigger the thyroid tissue, the higher the thyroglobulin. If the thyroid is inflamed, the value also increases. High values do not increase the risk for thyroid cancer. Before surgery, I usually do not measure it.

When do you measure thyroglobulin?

If you are confirmed to having thyroid cancer (papillary or follicular) after surgery and/or radioiodine ablation, we measure it to monitor thyroid cancer recurrence.

What is calcitonin?

Calcitonin is a hormone secreted by parafollicular cells (c cells) in response to increased calcium. The thyroid cancer derived from c cells is called medullary thyroid cancer. It is found in 3-5% of all thyroid cancers.

Should I have calcitonin checked in evaluating my Hashimoto's thyroiditis?

I do not recommend checking calcitonin routinely in evaluating Hashimoto's thyroiditis unless you have been suspected to have medullary thyroid cancer by biopsy, by family or personal history of MEN2, familial medullary thyroid cancer, or pheochromocytoma.

I also check calcitonin on patients who have a biopsy showing follicular lesions including Hurthle cell lesion.

Do I need to be fasting before a thyroid function test?

No, you do not need to be fasting for a thyroid function test.

Should I take my thyroid supplement on the day of testing?

Your total and free T4 and T3 might increase slightly for the first 4 hours after you take your medication. Your TSH will not be changed.

I recommend that my patients do whatever they usually do on the day of testing. No fasting and taking their medication as usual is recommended.

Some patients like to be fasting because they are accustomed. It is okay with me.

Chapter 3. Thyroid ultrasound and radioactive iodine uptake and scan

What does a normal thyroid ultrasound look like?

The normal thyroid is very smooth, and consistency is very good. It looks whiter than muscle. Here is my own thyroid ultrasound.

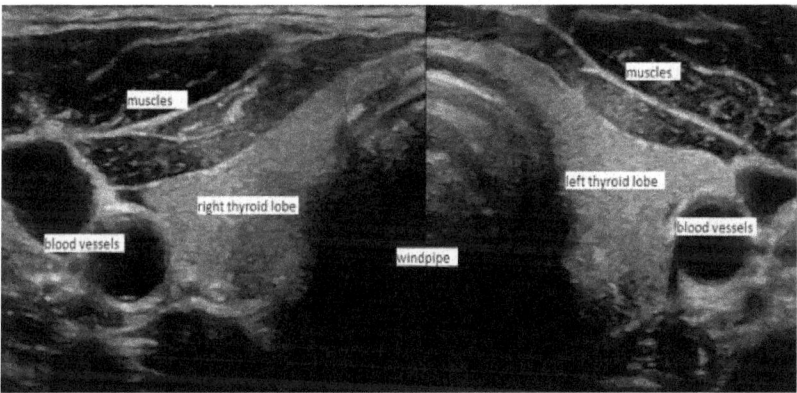

Figure. Normal thyroid ultrasound.

Should I have a thyroid ultrasound in evaluating Hashimoto's thyroiditis?

I recommend at least to have one thyroid ultrasound. Hashimoto's thyroiditis has specific features. Sometimes nodules concur with Hashimoto's thyroiditis. Some reports suggest that these nodules have increased risk for thyroid cancer.

If your thyroid function is not stable, I like to have a thyroid ultrasound to look at your stage of Hashimoto's thyroiditis and to see if anything else is going on such as thyroid nodules. If you have an overactive thyroid, then I definitely need to have a thyroid ultrasound. It can tell us the possible etiology of hyperthyroidism.

What are the typical features for Hashimoto's thyroiditis on thyroid ultrasound?

Hashimoto's thyroiditis is an evolving condition. At the different stages, the ultrasound can show the differences. Heterogeneity is a feature. Hypoechoic echogenicity (dark on the picture) is another feature. However, other conditions can cause heterogeneity such as subacute thyroiditis or amiodarone induced thyroiditis. The thyroid can be enlarged, normal, or small.

Sometimes there are benign-looking enlarged lymph nodes.

How do I prepare for a thyroid ultrasound exam?

You do not really need any preparation. I recommend wearing a low-cut shirt that makes the lower neck and thyroid area easily accessible.

Is there any harm to me?

We have not identified any harm or side effects for a thyroid ultrasound.

What is involved in a thyroid ultrasound exam?

We require you to lie flat and, if possible, to put a pillow under your shoulders to extend your neck.

Why are we doing thyroid scintigraphy (nuclear testing-usually called an iodine uptake and scan)?

Usually we do not need to have an iodine uptake and scan for diagnosing or managing Hashimoto's thyroiditis.

I recommend having iodine uptake and scan for the following situations:

- Patient has low TSH with or without nodules.
- Patient has overactive thyroid function test, but thyroid ultrasound does not show significant increased blood flow (vascularity).
- If you want to learn more about thyroid nodules. Please read my other book "Thyroid Nodules Questions from Real Patients".

What is the best isotope for thyroid scintigraphy?

I-123 is the most common isotope used for thyroid scintigraphy. The dose usually given is 200-400 uCi.

Does the radioactive iodine uptake and scan hurt my thyroid?

The dose used for iodine uptake and scan is very small. The effect on the thyroid is minimal and we only do it if you have an overactive thyroid, However, we do want to make sure you are not pregnant.

What precautions do I need to take after a radioactive iodine uptake and scan?

The dose is so small. You really do not need to take any precautions, but I recommend washing your hands well after using the bathroom and do not handle other people's food and drinks for two days. Do not stay close to a pregnant woman or an infant for two or three days. Do not have sex for three to four days.

Do I need to stay away from certain foods before the test?

One week before the test, I recommend staying off:
iodine vitamin supplements/iodized salt,

seaweed (kelp, etc), agar containing food, seafood (you might need to stay off longer), dairy products.

Do I need to stay away from certain medications before the test?

You need to stop:
- Antithyroid medication for one week
- Levothyroxine three to four weeks
- Triiodothyronine (Cytomel, T3) one to two weeks
- Topical iodine two to three weeks
- Amiodarone up to six months
- Avoid iodine contrast mediums for CT scans for six weeks to six months prior. Currently, with the commonly used contrast you usually need to wait two to six weeks.

Do I need to be fasting before the test?

You are recommended to fast eight hours before the test. However, two hours after you take the pill you are allowed to eat.

How is the test done?

- The test is usually performed at a nuclear department in a hospital.
- After taking the pill, you will be asked to be back in four hours and then the next day for the thyroid scan.
- The scan usually takes four to five minutes.

Can I have a PET scan for my Hashimoto's thyroiditis?

No, you do not need PET for diagnosis or managing Hashimoto's thyroiditis. I have many patients who are referred to me because they found PET scan signals in their thyroid. The PET was performed for other reasons.

It is well known that Hashimoto's thyroiditis can result in a PET scan signal. However, I will do a thyroid ultrasound to make sure there is no more than Hashimoto's thyroiditis.

When should I have a thyroid CT scan or MRI?

If your thyroid is so big that your doctor cannot get the full picture of your thyroid, a CT or MRI might be ordered to look at the thyroid size and the extension in relationship to surrounding structures, especially with retrosternal extension (extension in the chest). If a CT is ordered, usually non-contrast is recommended. High iodine in the contrast might cause hyperthyroidism.

Shunzhong Bao, MD

Chapter 4. Thyroid Hormone Replacement Therapy

What are our treatment goals?

We want to eliminate your symptoms and sign of hypothyroidism, to restore your sense of well-being, and to achieve normalcy in your thyroid function test.

For most patients, we do not know how to treat the causes yet but hormone replacement if patients have hypothyroidism. However, researches are underway to find the way how to treat the cause. Most researchers research IgG4 related Hashimoto's thyroiditis. Hopefully in the near future, we will have an easier way to diagnose IgG4 related Hashimoto's thyroiditis and treat it effectively and safely.

What is the side effect of thyroid hormone replacement?

All medication has side effects. Thyroid hormones are simple molecules. Your body should not be allergic to them, However, the pills you take have "fillers", so you might develop an allergy to them.

If you take too much, then you will develop symptoms of an "overactive thyroid", like palpitation, anxiety, restless, weight loss, etc.

If you take too much for a long time, it might cause osteoporosis and/or atrial fibrillation which increases your risk for a stroke.

What can we do to stop Hashimoto's thyroiditis?

Unfortunately, we still cannot stop the development of Hashimoto's thyroiditis. Your thyroid gland will evolve and change. In most cases, people will develop hypothyroidism, will need thyroid medication replacement, and eventually will need more and more medication over time.

Research is underway to stop the process of IgG4 related Hashimoto's thyroiditis with steroids and other immunosuppressants and have been reported to be very effective. However, without pathology, the diagnosis is difficult. The use of steroids and other immunosuppressants have many side effects, too.

Does taking thyroid hormones hurt my own thyroid gland?

Taking thyroid hormone is not hurting your own thyroid. It takes some pressure off your thyroid gland. It helps your thyroid gland, but most patients will not able to get off thyroid medications.

What is the rate of hypothyroidism (low thyroid) in Hashimoto's thyroiditis?

100% of all patients with Hashimoto's thyroiditis eventually will develop hypothyroidism, However, the process can be very long, like decades. Even when your doctor finds your thyroid function to be normal, you might still have periods of low thyroid. Why? Hashimoto's thyroiditis reduced your capacity to produce thyroid hormones. You need a different level of thyroid hormone at different times and lots of medications you take and food you eat might affect your thyroid production and T4 to T3 conversion (T3 is the active form of thyroid hormone).

I have patients with hyperthyroidism and gradually burn out to become hypothyroidism.

I also have patients who have had hypothyroidism for 40 years and suddenly converted to hyperthyroidism (overactive thyroid). For these patients, we usually recommend surgery or radioactive iodine to burn the thyroid. It is never a good idea to leave it alone and wait it to become hypothyroidism again.

The thyroid hormone is very important for your body to function properly, therefore the thyroid hormone needs to be replaced and the function test needs to be followed.

My thyroid function is normal. Do I need any treatment?

If your thyroid function is normal, theoretically you do not need any treatment. However, some researchers reported that selenium supplements are helpful. If you want to try, you can take selenium 200 ug daily. If you take too much of it, it can cause toxicity. You need to ask your doctor to check its level periodically.

From what medications for thyroid replacement can we choose from?

Currently we have the following medications from which you can choose to replace your thyroid hormone:
- Generic levothyroxine (T4)
- Levothroid (T4)
- Levoxyl (T4)

- Synthroid (T4)
- Unithyroid (T4)
- Tirosint (T4)
- Armour thyroid (T4+T3)
- Nature-throid(T4+T3)
- NP thyroid(T4+T3)
- WP-thyroid
- Cytomel (T3)
- Triostat (T3)
- Thyrolar (liotrix, T3+T4)

Which is best?

The most appropriate for you is the best.

How do you know what is the best for me?

While T4 formulation is generally recommended and most patients are doing very well in line with major professional society's recommendations, I am not afraid to use other non T4 formulations, like desiccated thyroid in combination with T4, or T3 alone or in combination with T4. I make decisions based on lab tests, but I do not disregard how patients feel. More importantly, I look into a patient's life and current medications because they are the major factors in interpreting the thyroid function tests.

What are the most commonly used medications in your clinic?

The most common one I use is generic levothyroxine. I also have a sizable number of patients on the brand names Synthroid and Levoxyl (which has been temporarily discontinued). Some patients are on Armour thyroid, Nature-throid, and NP thyroid. Only a few patients are on Tirosint and Cytomel. However, lately I recommend Tirosint-Sol more and more due to the clinical trial's report that the thyroid level can be achieved as stable as empty stomach while taking Tirosint-Sol immediately before food. However, the practice of taking your thyroid medication with food is still not recommended.

Is Synthroid (other brand names in other areas) better than generic?

Theoretically, brand name Synthroid is better. It is more stable since it is manufactured by one manufacturer. Generic levothyroxine is manufactured by many different manufacturers. Even if you get it from the same pharmacy, it may be coming from different manufacturers.

However, for most people the variations introduced are not because of the different manufacturers, it is because they take their medication at different times and may even forget to take it. The most important thing is to take thyroid medication consistently.

If your insurance pays for it or other brand names, I do not have a problem starting patients on Synthroid.

Can I take other brand names instead of Synthroid?

I do not have any problem starting my patients on any brand if their insurance pays for it. I have a few patients on Levoxyl but it has temporarily been discontinued. Synthroid is always present in my area of the country. Again, as I stated, I am using Tirosint-sol more and more.

Can I have an allergy to thyroid medication?

You should not be allergic to thyroid hormone itself but to the "fillers" of the pill.

What "fillers" are present in Synthroid?

Acacia, confectioner's sugar (contains corn starch), lactose monohydrate, magnesium stearate, povidone, and talc. Different doses of the medication also contain different coloring materials.

What is acacia? Could I be allergic to it?

Acacia is used to make the shape of the pill. It comes from shrubs and wood. Some people are allergic to it. If you have an allergy to tree pollens you might have an allergy to acacia, too.

I am lactose intolerant, and I saw Synthroid has lactose in it. Can I still take it?

The dose of lactose in the pill is very, very low. You should not have a problem taking it.

What is povidone? Is it toxic?

Povidone is a polymerized form of vinylpyrolidone, which is a white hygroscopic powder that is easily soluble in water and used as a dispersing and suspending agent in drugs like Synthroid. It seems safe and I have not seen any research about allergies to povidone. People can have a mild or severe allergy to povidone-iodine which is used as skin disinfectant.

What is talc? Is it cancer causing?

Talc is a naturally occurring mineral mined from the earth that is composed of magnesium, silicon, oxygen, and hydrogen. Chemically, talc is a hydrous magnesium silicate with a chemical formula of $Mg_3Si_4O_{10}(OH)_2$.

Talc has many uses in cosmetics and other personal care products; in food such as rice and chewing gum; and in the manufacturing of tablets.

The cousin of talc-asbestos is a cancer-causing agent. There is no evidence to show that talc causes cancer or allergies.

Synthroid comes in different colors. What are the color agents in the pill?

Synthroid has 12 different strengths (mcg) with 12 different colors.

Table. Synthroid tablet color and additives.

Strength (mcg)	Color additive(s)
25	orange--FD&C Yellow No. 6 Aluminum Lake
50	white------None
75	violet----FD&C Red No. 40 Aluminum Lake, and FD&C Blue No. 2 Aluminum Lake
88	olive------FD&C Blue No. 1 Aluminum Lake, FD&C Yellow No. 6 Aluminum Lake, D&C Yellow No. 10 Aluminum Lake
100	yellow---D&C Yellow No. 10 Aluminum Lake, FD&C Yellow No. 6 Aluminum Lake

112	rose--D&C Red No. 27 & 30 Aluminum Lake
125	brown-FD&C Yellow No. 6 Aluminum Lake, FD&C Red No. 40 Aluminum Lake, FD&C Blue No. 1 Aluminum Lake
137	Turquoise-FD&C Blue No. 1 Aluminum Lake
150	blue-FD&C Blue No. 2 Aluminum Lake
175	lilac-FD&C Blue No. 1 Aluminum Lake, D&C Red No. 27 & 30 Aluminum Lake
200	pink-FD&C Red No. 40 Aluminum Lake
300	green-D&C Yellow No. 10 Aluminum Lake, FD&C Yellow No. 6 Aluminum Lake, FD&C Blue No. 1 Aluminum Lake

Is aluminum lake toxic?

Aluminum lake is aluminum oxide. It is believed to be nontoxic.

Can I have an allergy to dyes?

Yes, it is possible. If suspected, you can try the dosage of 50 ug which does not have coloring agents. I use this as a base to make different doses. The following is my scheme to make different doses.

- 25 ug: ½ tab daily

- 50 ug: 1 tab daily
- 75 ug: 1 and ½ tabs daily
- 88 ug: 5 days of 2 tabs daily, and 2 days of 1 tab daily
- 100 ug: 2 tabs daily
- 112 ug: 6 days of 2 tabs daily and one day of 3.5 tabs.
- 125 ug: 2.5 tabs daily
- 137 ug: 3 tabs daily for 6 days and 1 tab for one day.
- 150 ug: 3 tabs daily
- 175 ug: 3.5 tabs daily
- 200 ug: 4 tabs daily
- 250 ug: 5 tabs daily
- 300 ug: 6 tabs daily

Why are colors added to the pills?

I have no ideal. I think the manufacturers might want to help patients to identify the pills because there are so many different dosese.

What is the color scheme for other T4 brands?

Most of them use the same color scheme, but there are some differences.

Table. The color scheme of other T4 brands

Strength (ug)	Levothroid (Actavis)	Levoxyl (Pfizer)	Synthroid (Abbvie)	Unithroid (Watson)
25	orange	orange	orange	peach
50	white	white	white	white
75	violet	purple	violet	purple
88	mint green	olive	olive	olive
100	yellow	yellow	yellow	yellow
112	rose	rose	rose	rose

125	brown	brown	brown	tan
137	deep blue	dark blue	turquoise	Not available
150	blue	blue	blue	blue
175	lilac	turquoise	lilac	lilac
200	pink	pink	pink	pink
300	green	green	green	green

Is Tirosint better?

It is believed that Tirosint, especially Tirosint-Sol has better absorption. Patients with atrophic gastritis, patients taking anti-acid medications, or patients with a history of gastric bypass surgery could benefit from this due to absorption issues. I do not worry about this too much, I usually just increase the dose. If your insurance will pay for it and you believe it works better for you, I do not have a problem prescribing it.

I have patients who have malabsorption and I have prescribed 500-1000 ug of levothyroxine. I wanted to try Tirosint but was not able to get insurance to pay for it. When the coverage becomes better, I will prescribe Tirosint-Sol or Tirosint soft gel more and more. I think in near term the generic levothyroxine solution/liquid will be available.

What fillers does Tirosint have?

Inactive ingredients: gelatin, glycerin, and water.
People might have an allergic reaction to gelatin, but usually not to glycerin. Certainly if you do have allergic to glycerin, then you can not take it.

What fillers does Tirsosint-Sol have?

Tirosint-Sol only have T4, water and glycerin. Tirosint-Sol only has glycerin as the "filler".

Do you think the new released doses of Tirosint are helpful for your patients?

Now Tirosint gel and Tirosint-Sol have three more extra doses: 37.5, 44 and 62.5 mcg. In my opinion, the dose of 62.5 mcg is very useful. I have many patients who are taking the dose of 50 mcg and 75 mcg alternatively. Sometimes, patients are confused and have to pay two prescription copays. Now they do not have to do that. The dose of 37.5 mcg and 44 mcg are not that useful. Maybe they will be helpful if we have patients who need slightly less than the dose of 50 mcg. I have not prescribed these two doses yet.

Does Tirosint have color coding?

No, Tirosint does not have color coding on the gel. If you are allergic to color agents, this version might be a good option for you. However, if your insurance doesn't pay for it or it is too expensive for you, you can use my scheme to form a different dosage with colorless 50 ug pills.

On the boxes, the color coding is as follows.

Strength (ug)	Color on the box
13	green
25	peach

37.5	dark blue
44	red
50	white
62.5	gray
100	purple
112	yellow
125	brown
150	blue

Does Tirosint cause less allergic reactions?

Yes. Tirosint has fewer fillers and no coloring agents added. If you are looking for "pure" thyroid hormone replacement, this is the purest.

I have patients who also have claimed to have an allergic reaction to it. Presumably they are allergic to gelatin. Many vaccines also have gelatin. If you are allergic to vaccines then you might be allergic to Tirosint. but vaccines have more allergens in them.

Now if you think you are allergic to Tirosint gel we can try Tirosint-Sol which only has glycerin.

How are Tirosint capsules supplied?

They are supplied as follows: boxes of 56 capsules, consisting of 8 blisters with 7 capsules each.

What is the best time to take T4 formulations like generic levothyroxine, Synthroid, Levoxyl, Levothroid, Unithroid, or Tirosint?

It is recommended to take them early in the morning on an empty stomach, ideally 60 minutes before you drink anything except water, eat, or take any other medications.

However, most of my patients are not able to do that. I usually ask my patients to put the medication and a cup of water on their nightstand the night before and, as soon as they open their eyes, pop in the medication with a cup of water. During the night, you lose a lot of water, so it is good for you to drink a cup of water when you wake up.

Can I take T4 formulations like generic levothyroxine, Synthroid, Levoxyl, Levothroid, Unithroid, or Tirosint at night?

I have patients who cannot take it early in the morning, so I ask them to take it before going to bed. I urge them to not eat any snacks after dinner. Bedtime and dinner should be at least four hours apart.

How do I take Tirosint soft gel?

You should take it as other levothyroxine preparations.

How do I take Tirosint-Sol?

You can take it by squeeze the liquid directly into your month. It recommended that you squeeze five times until no liquid coming out of it. Then I recommended you following up with a glass of water. I still recommended that you do not eat or take other medications for ½ to one hours after. There are clinical researches reported that eating immediately after taking Tirosint-Sol does not affect the absorption significantly. However, this practice is still not recommended.

What should I do if I forget a day?

It is best not to forget, but life happens, so if you forget, I recommend you double it the next day.

Do you have any options for my son who is 16 years old? He never remembers to take his meds and I cannot be after him every day to take them.

Your son is not alone. Lots of teens are not good at taking medications. They either forget, do not want to take it, or wake up too late. It is very challenging for teens to take thyroid medication.

I recommend my patients to choose one day each week and to take seven pills all at once. It is not ideal but at least you know they consistently get taken.

I have malabsorption. What options do I have?

Tirosint may be better for you if your insurance will pay for it. Otherwise, I would just increase your dose.

However, I have patients who have such severe malabsorption that we must give intravenous levothyroxine periodically and insurance usually will balk at paying for it.

I have Crohn's disease. Do you have any recommendations for me?

Crohn's disease is an inflammatory bowel disease. It can be very challenging with flair ups and changes in absorption rates in the body. You can try Tirosint which has a better absorption rate. The key issue is to check your thyroid function more often.

I am also taking iron and calcium supplements. Any extra precautions?

Iron and calcium affect thyroid medication absorption significantly. I recommend you take your calcium or iron pills at least four hours after taking your thyroid medication. If you take your thyroid medication in the morning, then I recommend you take iron or calcium at supper or at night.

I am also taking an osteoporosis medication called bisphosphonates-like Actonel (risedronate), Fosamax (alendronate), Boniva (ibandronate), Pamidronate. Can I take my thyroid hormone with these medications?

These medications also require you to take them early in the morning on an empty stomach and then wait 60 minutes before you eat or drink anything else except water.

Since these medications are usually taken once a week or once a month, I am not particularly worried about these.
If you take your thyroid medication and osteoporosis medication together it might affect your thyroid medication absorption. Since T4 formulations (generic levothyroxine, Synthroid, Levoxyl, Levothroid,

45

Unithroid, or Tirosint) come with half-life of seven days, one day of lower absorption will not affect your blood thyroid level too much. Your thyroid hormone level will be stable.

If you do not want to take them together, you can also omit your thyroid hormone on the day you are taking the bisphosphonates and then double up your thyroid medication the next day.

However, if you are newly starting your bisphosphonates, I recommend having your thyroid function checked in six weeks and adjusting your dose as needed.

I am also taking acid reflux / stomach medications, H pump inhibitors like Nexium (esomeprazole), Omeprazole, Pantoprazole, Lansoprazole, Dexilant (dexlansoprazole), or Aciphex (rabeprazole) medications. My doctors tell me to take them on an empty stomach. What should I do?

These medications might reduce thyroid medication absorption, but most studies say NO. The good news is that your doctor can always increase the thyroid medication dose as needed. I first let my patients take their thyroid medication with these medications together on an empty stomach to see if we can get their thyroid level stable.

Another option is to take the thyroid medication at night. However, these patients are also taking other medications at night which might affect their thyroid medication absorption. It is better to take them together in the morning.

I have patients who like to take thyroid medication 30 minutes before taking these mentioned medications. This option is also acceptable. The key issue is consistency.

Certainly, if you start later you will need to check your thyroid function in 4-6 weeks after you are started on H pump inhibitors to make sure you are taking sufficient thyroid medication.

I am taking antacids, what should I pay attention to?

If you are taking antacids like aluminum hydroxide, magnesium hydroxide, Alka-seltzer, Pepto, Maalox, Mylanta (aluminum hydroxide/magnesium hydroxide), Rolaids, or Tums, these medications should be taken at least four hours after thyroid medication. I strongly recommend you take your thyroid medication early in the morning on an empty stomach with a cup of room temperature or warm water.

I am taking carafate for my stomach ulcer. I heard this medication can affect thyroid medication absorption. What should I do?

It is true that carafate reduces thyroid medication absorption. This medication might be taken four times a day and needs to be taken one hour before a meal. In this situation, I recommend taking your thyroid medication 30 minutes before taking carafate with a cup of warm water. Close monitoring and adjusting thyroid medication is strongly recommended.

What other medications should I pay attention to while taking thyroid medication?

If you are taking any of the following medications, you should take them at least four hours apart from thyroid medication. Consistency is the key. Let your thyroid doctor know so the dose can be adjusted:

- Cholestyramine-cholesterol medication.
- Colesevelam--cholesterol medication.
- Selevemer-lower phosphorus in renal failure patients.

- Raloxifene (Evista)-breast cancer prevention and treating osteoporosis.

There are certainly many other medications which might affect thyroid medication absorption. Keep taking the medications four hours apart if you can.

I was told that I cannot take my thyroid medication with coffee. However, I always rush in the morning. There is no way that I can wait 60 minutes before I drink my coffee. Are you sure I absolutely cannot drink coffee?

Life is complicated as you described and taking thyroid medication certainly makes it more complicated. I am very liberal. If you are willing to promise that you drink the same coffee at same time every day, I will let you try. We can always adjust your thyroid medication dose.

Another option is to take your thyroid medication at night. After dinner you are not supposed to eat snacks for at least four hours.

I cannot wait 60 minutes before I eat my breakfast. What should I do?

Milk and soy products, coffee and other fibers all affect thyroid medication absorption. As I recommended, prepare a cup of water on your nightstand the night before. As soon as you open your eyes, pop in your thyroid medication. After you get washed and dressed, 30 minutes might have passed. This is not 60 minutes as recommended, but it will be acceptable.

I also have patients taking their thyroid medication when they wake up in the middle of night or early morning. You are allowed to take it at that time.

If you do not eat snack at night, then taking at night can be an option for you to try as long as you can take it four hours after your last meal or snack.

Another option is taking Tirosint-Sol. Although it is not recommended to eat immediately after you take Tirosint-Sol, there are reports that in doing so, the levels of T4 and TSH do not change significantly.

Whatever you do, if you can do it consistently it is not a big deal. We can always adjust your dose.

How do you decide which dose to start?

I use the information of the patient's weight, lean body mass, pregnancy status, cause of hypothyroidism (RAI or surgery), degree of TSH elevation, age, history of cardiovascular disease, and other conditions including the presence of cardiac disease. The most important thing is to have follow up and adjust your medication. It is very important to start right, but more important is to adjust and take your medication correctly and consistently.

I swear that I feel better when I am on Armour thyroid. My former endocrinologist did not believe me. Do you believe me?

I believe you, and I have 20% of my patients who like to take a desiccated thyroid product like Armour thyroid.

The thyroid gland is complicated. The thyroid gland secretes a variety of iodinated and non-iodinated molecules that collectively play important roles during our prenatal and adult lives. We do not understand them yet. When I was an Endocrine Fellow at Washington University School of Medicine, I had a fellow classmate who did research on calcitonin. He claimed that replacement of calcitonin affects feelings of wellbeing.

My approach to this request is to keep an open mind. I acknowledged that a T4 formulation like levothyroxine is the mainstream supplement and it is very easy to take. Most patients are doing very well on this. I let patients try other formulations if they are not happy about their current medication. I do let patients know that there are many reasons which might cause them to not feel well that we cannot fix with thyroid medications. I also let my patients know that sometimes we will have to use desiccated thyroid two times a day due to high levels of T3 in it. The dose difference between each batch may be larger even from the same manufacturer, and sometimes it is very difficult to have a right dose. Also the T4, T3 and other molecules might vary from batch to batch. Desiccated thyroid also has a lab test that is sometimes difficult for a non-specialist to interpret.

The manufacturer also advises that a potential risk of product contamination with porcine and bovine viral or other adventitious agents cannot be ruled out.

What is Armour thyroid anyway?

Armour Thyroid for oral use is a natural preparation derived from porcine thyroid glands. They provide 38 mcg levothyroxine (T4) and 9 mcg liothyronine (T3) per grain of thyroid (equivalent of 60 mg).

What is WP thyroid or Nature-throid?

They are two other products from desiccated pig thyroid. I treat them the same as Armour thyroid, however the dose forms are slightly different.

What is the dose equivalent between desiccated thyroid and T4 preparations like levothyroxine?

Usually, I start 100 ug of levothyroxine converted to 60 mg (grain) of Armour thyroid or 65 mg (grain) of WP thyroid or Nature-throid.

The Armour thyroid and NP thyroid has a dose increment of 15 mg (equivalent to levothyroxine 25 ug).

The WP thyroid and Nature-throid have dose increments of 16.25 mg equivalent to levothyroxine 25 ug.

What are the inactive ingredients in the pill?

The inactive ingredients are calcium stearate, dextrose, microcrystalline cellulose, sodium starch glycolate, and opadry white.

Can I have an allergy to natural desiccated thyroid?

Yes, you can.

How do I know if I am allergic to Armour thyroid or other desiccated thyroid supplements?

Allergic reactions can include the following but are not limited to rashes, hives, itching, difficulty breathing, tightness in the chest, swelling of the mouth, face, lips or tongue.

When it happens, you certainly need to stop the medication. If you have mild symptoms like a rash or itching, you can just take antihistamine medications like Benadryl. If you have problems like difficulty breathing, tightness in the chest, swelling of the mouth, face, lips or tongue, do not waste your time calling your doctor's office. Go to the ER immediately.

Shunzhong Bao, MD

Can I take my Armour thyroid or other desiccated thyroid at night?

Theoretically it is okay to take it at night. The thyroid effect in cells needs a few hours to work. However, I still have patients complaining about it affecting their sleep. My point is that you can try it and if it does not affect your sleep, you can take it at bedtime.

Table of the dose conversions between commonly used thyroid replacement preparation.

Levothyroxine Mcg	Armour grain(mg)	WP thyroid grain(mg)	Nature-throid grain(mg)
25	¼(15)	¼(16.25) ¼(16.25)	
50	½(30)	½(32.5)	½(32.5)
75		¾(48.75)	¾(48.75)
88			
100	1(60)	1(65)	1(65)
112			
125		1.25(81.25)	1/25(81.25)
137			
150	1.5(90)	1.5(97.5)	1.5(97.5)
175		1.75(113.75)	1.75(113.75)
200	2(120)	2(130)	2(130)
			2.25(146.25)
			2.5(162.5)
300	3(180)		3.0(195)
	4(240)		4(260)
	5(300)		5(325)

Please note this is just a starting point. Everybody is different. You need to have close monitor your thyroid function and get your dose adjusted accordingly.

I am on a thyroid supplement. Do I need to take extra iodine?

No, you do not. You already are being supplemented with an iodine product of the thyroid hormone.

I am on a thyroid supplement. Do I need to take a selenium supplement?

Selenium helps you to convert T4 to the active hormone T3. However, most people do not have a selenium deficiency and you might not need to take it. If you want to take it, it is acceptable, and it might help you. However, if you take too much, it can cause toxicity.

My TSH is low. Why did my doctor reduce my thyroid medication?

As we discussed previously, TSH is like a thermostat. If your thyroid hormone level is too high, then TSH is going to be reduced. The opposite is true also. If your thermostat ramps up it means the temperature at your house is too low. If the TSH is too high it means your thyroid hormone level is too low. That is why when your TSH is low your doctor will lower your thyroid medication; if your TSH is too high, your doctor will increase your medication.

Just remember, the TSH level is always opposite to your thyroid hormone level. The premise is that you have a normal pituitary gland.

I heard that taking thyroid medication can help me to lose weight. Can I take more?

It is really a bad idea to take more thyroid medication to lose weight. Too much thyroid medication may cause atrial fibrillation which will increase your risk for stroke. Too much thyroid medication can also cause osteoporosis. These are the two most serious side effects.

Why is my FT4 always elevated and TSH is normal?

This usually occurs with the following situation:
Most patients are being treated with T4 (levothyroxine, Synthroid, Levoxyl, etc). The medication usually is being absorbed within 4 hours and can have a peek in the blood. If you check your blood 2-4 hours after you take your medication, your blood value of T4 might be higher than normal.

Do I need to reduce my dose if FT4 is high?

No, I adjust your medication based on many factors. As we can see from the above question, T4 will have a peak in 2-4 hours after taking the medication. You certainly do not need to reduce your medication if this is the case. I usually look at the full panel of thyroid function and your symptoms and signs. If your TSH is suppressed and you have some signs of overactive thyroid, certainly we need to reduce your dose.

My FT3 is always low. What are the reasons?

Assuming your TSH and FT4 are normal, here are some reasons:
- Your Hashimoto's thyroiditis is at the end stage, which means your thyroid doesn't work at all. Since the thyroid is responsible to produce 20% of T3, now you do not have it.

- You might be taking some medications which can suppress deiodinase which is the enzyme responsible to convert T4 to T3.
- You might have low activity of deiodinase gene function.

What are the medications that might inhibit the function of deiodinase?

There is a long list medication which might inhibit the conversion of T4 to T3. Here are a few common medications:
- Steroids
- Beta blocker, especially propranolol. Other commonly used beta blockers are atenolol, metoprolol, labetalol, and Coreg.
- Amiodarone (medication for irregular heartbeat) can cause a range of thyroid problems.
- Lithium (mood stabilizer) can cause a spectrum of thyroid issues.

What are common conditions which might inhibit the function of deiodinase?

Some conditions and disease status can also inhibit deiodinase, reducing T4 to T3 conversion:
- Very sick
- Lots of stress
- Lots of inflammation
- Starvation/deprivation
- Selenium deficiency

What can I do if my T3 is low?

There are many options. I make decisions depending on the patient's clinical comorbidities and symptoms. If the patient is relatively healthy, their TSH is still normal, but still has lots of hypothyroidism symptoms, I might increase your thyroid medication dose, or add a low dose T3 into your regimen. If you are not on "desiccated thyroid", I might let you try.

My doctor changes my dose every time I have my lab test. What should I do?

You are not alone. I have quite a few patients who are referred to me for unstable thyroid. The level is up and down. They have tried every dose of thyroid medication. I recommend you see a specialist like me (Endocrinologist).

I take my medication everyday consistently. Why does my thyroid level still change every time I have a lab test?

Hashimoto's thyroiditis is a chronic autoimmune inflammatory disease. It is an ongoing destructive and repairing process. It is expected to have unstable thyroid function tests for very severe patients especially with goiter and a severe swing of symptoms, after we try different T4 formulations and other measures, we have to recommend thyroidectomy or radioactive iodine treatment.

Both you and your doctor should realize that the nature of your Hashimoto's thyroiditis might cause your thyroid function to fluctuate.

I have had hypothyroidism (underactive thyroid) treated with thyroid medication for 40 years, and now my doctor said that I have hyperthyroidism (overactive thyroid). Is this possible?

The exact cause and disease process are not very clear yet. As we discussed, some patients have two kinds of antibodies. One antibody can block the thyrotropin receptor and then cause hypothyroidism

(Hashimoto's thyroiditis), and one antibody can stimulate the thyrotropin receptor and then cause hyperthyroidism (overactive thyroid, Hashimoto's thyrotoxicosis). I have quite a few patients like you who have had long standing hypothyroidism that converted to hyperthyroidism. In this case, I just treat as hyperthyroidism. Eventually I treated them with surgery or radioactive iodine.

My labs are in the normal range, but I still feel cold and dry skin. Can I increase my dose?

It depends on your clinical situation. These symptoms are nonspecific and not very sensitive to adjusting your dose. However, if your lab results are still in the normal range, I might increase your dose to let you raise your thyroid hormone level to the midpoint and up to a third of the normal range.

Chapter 5. My lab test is good, but I do not feel well (13 cases).

The thyroid is more complicated than we thought. Our body is more complicated than we thought. Life is more complicated than we thought

More things are happening in the thyroid or related to the thyroid, but we do not know how to measure them.

More things are happening in our body that we still do not know.

More things are happening in our life that we consciously or unconsciously do not appreciate.

I am going to share with you some of the cases referred to me with normal thyroid function, but they did not feel well.

Case 1. 35-year-old female presented with normal TSH and tied of being tired.

A 35-year-old female was referred to me for fatigue. It turned out that she had a very complicated past medical history and sad story. She was married to her high school sweetheart at the age of 19 and had a son at the age of 20. She lost her job at age 25 and was divorced at age 26. Now she is 35 and on disability.

She has been visiting our local hospitals numerous times for acute shortness of breath. She was diagnosed with idiopathic heart failure, and she was put on the heart transplant waiting list. She came to me partly because she heard that not feeling could be due to a hormonal problem like a thyroid or an adrenal problem.

The first time I saw her she was really in a depressed mood. Who wouldn't be? No job, and on the heart transplant waiting list, she could die at any time. She looked ill, and pale. She was also complained of no energy at all, dry skin and hair loss, no sex drive and no desire to date or, as a matter of fact, to do anything. She came to me just because she was tired of being so tired.

It turned out that when she gave birth to her son at age of 20 she had pretty severe bleeding and received a few units of blood. After the birth, she did not have enough milk and then she put her son on formula. She had been tired all the time. As a mother with a job and a husband, she was thinking she should have been tired. A few years before she went to the ER and received her a diagnosis of heart failure. She had more reasons to be tired and not feeling well.

We checked her thyroid function. Her TSH was 0.7 which was normal. However, her FT3 and FT4 were both low. She had her thyroid function was checked and was told it was normal. The reason is that only TSH was checked, not the full panel of thyroid function. Even the FT3 and FT4 were checked sometimes in the ER department, and doctors just assumed that they were low due to a non-thyroidal illness.

She actually also had very low sex hormones and adrenal hormone.

What is the diagnosis?

The diagnosis: Hypopituitarism/Sheehan's syndrome.

What is the Sheehan's syndrome?

Sheehan's syndrome is a form of hypopituitarism caused by pituitary infarction, which is caused by severe postpartum hemorrhaging (bleeding).

How is the diagnosis of Sheehan's syndrome made?

The patient needs to have a history of severe postpartum hemorrhaging. She also needed to have a history and evidence of hypopituitarism. We will check every pituitary hormone.

What are other reasons for hypopituitarism?

There are many reasons which can cause hypopituitarism. If you suspect that you might have hypopituitarism, you need to see an endocrinologist.

Here are a few reasons:
- Pituitary tumor or other tumor too close to the pituitary with or without surgery

- Traumatic brain injury (TBI)
- Infarction
- Some autoimmune disease
- Some infiltrative disease (see case two)
- Brain radiation
- Infection

How do we treat hypopituitarism?

We supplement with those end gland deficient hormones. We usually treat with end gland like thyroid hormones T4 or T3, not pituitary hormone TSH. In her case, we treated with levothyroxine. We treated with steroids instead of pituitary hormone ACTH. In her case, we treated with hydrocortisone. We treated with sex hormones instead of pituitary hormones FSH or LH. She was started on OCP (oral contraceptives). These are the most critical hormones.

Growth hormone can be replaced, but it is not very crucial.

For possible diabetes insipidus, we usually treat with DDAVP, a synthetic antidiuretic hormone. Most people do not need it. She did not need it.

Outcome of my patient:

After nine months of treatment, her heart is back to normal and she is off the heart transplant list. She went back to the workforce and she has been trying to reclaim her life. Last time I saw her five years ago she was dating and very happy.

Case 2: 35-year-old male presented with 20 years of diabetes insipidus.

This patient was technically not referred to me because of abnormal thyroid. However, he is another case of normal TSH and the treating physician thought his thyroid was normal. He was not feeling well. He was referred to me because he was suspected to have diabetes insipidus. Diabetes insipidus is different from diabetes mellitus. It is a over-urination and water-drinking problem.

He was referred to see me at age 35 for diabetes insipidus. The real story went back to age 15. Since that time, he has always felt thirsty and drank a few gallons of water a day. He went to the bathroom 4-10 times. I do not know how he got any sleep. He also had periods of headaches every night. Sometimes the headache was better and sometimes it was worse. Amazingly, he developed normally and was able to find a job and got married. Unfortunately, he was not able to hold his job due to severe fatigue that also affected his marriage. Eventually he lost his job and was divorced.

On physical examination, I found a yellowish skin patch in between his eyes. I saw one similar case when I was an endocrinology fellow at Washington University School of Medicine. I suspected that he might have infiltrative disease. His headache MRI indeed revealed a gigantic tumor-like structure. I referred him to a neurosurgeon at Washington University and he had a biopsy which revealed xanthogranuloma.

What is xanthogranuloma?

In our defense system, we have a group of cells called macrophages. They were so named because they are very big compared to other cells and they also do the job of "invader eater". "Phage" means eater in Greek.

Xanthogranuloma is a disease of macrophages. It is not cancer but like cancer grows too much. They can infiltrate the skin forming patches of rash on the skin and they can infiltrate the pituitary and cause hypopituitarism.

How do we make the diagnosis?

The diagnosis is based on a biopsy. My patient actually had two biopsies, the skin biopsy and brain biopsy. Both were confirmed xanthogranuloma.

What is the cause for xanthogranuloma?

We still do not know.

How do we treat xanthogranuloma?

This condition is not cancer but behaves like cancer. It is treated like cancer. My patient was treated with chemotherapy, and radiation.

His pituitary hormone was also replaced. In his case, we treated with steroids, thyroid hormone, and testosterone. He was also treated with DDAVP for diabetes insipidus.

What is the outcome of your patient?

He battled with this disease for three years, but he won!
Now his headaches are absolutely gone.
His adrenal function was recovered, and he no longer needs any steroids. His antidiuretic hormone has also recovered, and he does not need DDAVP anymore. He is still on thyroid medication and testosterone.

He reclaimed his life. Now he is in his last year of a radiology technician program. He is full of energy and lost significant weight. He is not ready to date yet, but the bottom-line is that he is very happy.

Case 3. 48-year-old female presented with Hashimoto's thyroiditis and unrelieved fatigue

This is a 48-year-old female. She was referred for "not feeling well". She was diagnosed with Hashimoto's thyroiditis 15 years ago. She has tried all different thyroid medications - like Synthroid and Armour thyroid. She was taking Armour thyroid. Her thyroid function was essentially normal. Her TSH was normal and FT3 was normal. FT4 was slightly low. She still continued to gain weight, was always tired, and losing hair. This is why she was finally referred to Endocrinologist. Her doctor hoped I could do better for her thyroid.

I received a detailed history. I noticed that she still had her menstrual periods, but they were very irregular and sometimes very heavy.

Her blood count was slightly low. However, her iron was low, and her iron saturation was very low. She had severe iron deficiency anemia.

What is iron deficiency?

Iron plays a very important role in our body. It is not just needed for making blood. It also plays very important roles in other body functions and processes. Iron is very important for myoglobin to work. Myoglobin is the major protein of muscles and is responsible for muscle contraction. Iron is also important for cell respiratory chains (our body uses this chain to break down carbs and fat to make the energy our body can use readily). Iron is very important for catalase. Catalase is an enzyme to break down the peroxide in our body. If peroxide is not broken down it will kill a lot of cells used to kill bacteria.

What are the symptoms of iron deficiency?

Iron deficiency can cause all the symptoms hypothyroidism can cause. Thyroid hormone is very important for every cell to work properly. Iron is also very important for cells to work properly.

People with iron deficiency can have symptoms like fatigue, weakness, exercise intolerance, not feeling well, depression, headaches, irritability, and if severe enough, shortness of breath, and chest pain.

People with iron deficiency also frequently have dry skin, dry nails, cracked nails, loss of hair, and dry hair.

People with iron deficiency also complain of poor memory and also like to eat ice.

People with iron deficiency can have something called **beeturia**. Beeturia is a phenomenon in which the urine turns red following ingestion of beets.

Beeturia is caused by increased intestinal absorption and subsequent excretion of the reddish pigment betalaine (betanin) present in beets. Betalaine, a redox indicator, is decolorized by ferric ions, which presumably explains the predisposition to beeturia when adequate amounts of iron are not available for decolorization of this pigment.

How do we diagnosis iron deficiency?

It is very easy to diagnose iron deficiency. You just need to check the iron panel: your iron, iron binding capacity, percentage of iron binding capacity and ferritin.

Making the diagnosis of iron deficiency is step 1. Step 2 is to find the cause. This is very important to resolve the problem.

What are the common causes for iron deficiency?

- The most common cause is blood loss, especially for women during their reproductive age. Excessive blood loss from heavy menstrual periods is the most common cause.
- Any men or postmenopausal women with iron deficiency deserve to have a further gastrointestinal (GI) workup.
- Hashimoto's thyroiditis patients also have higher risk for food allergy or celiac disease which can also cause iron deficiency.
- These days, we have too many people who take anti-acid medication. Iron is dependent on the acid being absorbed.
- If you have gastric bypass or other GI tract surgery, in my opinion, checking your iron level is mandatory.
- Patients are taking blood thinner.

What are the oral formulations?

For most patients, we have to use an oral form first. However, I found lots of patients cannot tolerate them due to severe constipation. They may be ineffective because many patients are taking anti-acid medications.

The following are a few frequently used products:

- Ferrous sulfate
  - Some brand names: BProtected Pedia Iron [OTC]; Fer-In-Sol [OTC]; Fer-Iron [OTC] [DSC]; FeroSul [OTC];Ferro-Bob [OTC]; FerrouSul [OTC]; Iron Supplement Childrens [OTC];Slow Fe [OTC];Slow Iron [OTC]
  - 325 mg tablet (contains 65 mg elemental iron per tablet)
  - 220 mg/5 mL oral elixir (contains 44 mg elemental iron per 5 mL)
  - 75 mg/mL oral solution (contains 15 mg elemental iron per mL)
- Ferrous gluconate
  - Fergon: 240 mg [elemental iron 27 mg] [DSC] [contains tartrazine (fd&c yellow #5)]
  - Generic: 240 mg [elemental iron 27 mg], 324 mg [elemental iron 38 mg]
    Tablet, Oral [preservative free]:
  - Ferate: 240 mg [elemental iron 27 mg] [corn free, dairy free, egg free, fragrance free, gluten free, no artificial flavor(s), sodium free, soy free, starch free, sugar free, wheat free, yeast free; contains fd&c blue #1 aluminum lake, fd&c yellow #6 aluminum lake]
  - Ferate: 256 mg [elemental iron 28 mg] [DSC] [gluten free, lactose free, milk free, no artificial color(s), no

artificial flavor(s), sodium free, soy free, sugar free, wheat free, yeast free]
  - o Generic: 324 mg [elemental iron 37.5 mg]
- Ferrous fumarate
  - o Ferretts: 325 mg (106 mg elemental iron) [scored]
  - o Ferrimin 150: Elemental iron 150 mg
  - o Ferrocite: 324 mg (106 mg elemental iron) [DSC] [contains fd&c blue #1 aluminum lake, fd&c yellow #5 aluminum lake]
  - o Hemocyte: 324 mg (106 mg elemental iron)
  - o Generic: 90 mg (29.5 mg elemental iron) [DSC], 324 mg (106 mg elemental iron),
- Polysaccharide-iron complex and folic acid
  Solution

  - o NovaFerrum®: Elemental iron 100 mg and folic acid 1 mg per 5 mL (120 mL [DSC]) [contains ascorbic acid 60 mg/5 mL; raspberry-grape flavor]
  Capsule

  - o EZFE 200, Ferrex 150, Ferric-X 150, iFerex 150, Myferon 150, NovaFerrum 50, Nu-Iron 150, PIC 200, Poly-Iron 150

Which oral formulation is the best?

I don't know which one is the best. Sometimes, I recommend Slow-iron. It seems to be better tolerated. However, the rate of absorption is low. I prefer to refer my patients to have iron infusions which I believe provides the best and quickest results. Some patients use Integra (ferrous fumarate, polysaccharide iron, vitamin C and niacin) and have good results. Some patients reported that ferrous bisglycinate or diglycinate are better tolerated

How should I take the oral iron supplement?

Since iron affects thyroid medication absorption you should not take iron and thyroid medication together. Lots of medications and foods also affect iron absorption.

I recommend taking one tab/capsule/or liquid at bedtime. Ideally your meal is four hours before bedtime. Snacking is not recommended. Take one a day or every other day if you are not tolerating it very well. Studies show that every other day may be even better. Therefore, iron is not recommended to be taken two to three times a day.

I also recommend my patients to take 250 mg of vitamin C with the iron especially if they are taking anti-acid medications.

What food and medications can affect the iron absorption significantly?

Calcium supplements are the most common medications which can severely affect iron absorption. Any high fiber food, cereal, milk and milk containing products, tea, coffee, and eggs all affect iron absorption.

Drinking too much tea actually can cause iron deficiency.

How long should I take my iron supplement?

If your cause for iron deficiency is corrected, then you just need to get your iron to normal and you do not need to continue. However, if your cause is not known or cannot be corrected, then you have to take it all the time.

What are the side effects of oral iron supplements?

Gastrointestinal side effects are extremely common with oral iron administration. Most patients have constipation already. The iron supplement is not welcomed by patients. Other side effects are metallic taste, nausea, flatulence, diarrhea, epigastric distress, and/or vomiting. Patients may also be bothered by itching and by black/green or tarry stools that stain clothing or cause anxiety about bleeding.

What can we do if oral iron is not tolerated?

I am a big fan of intravenous iron supplement. It is fast and effective. Most patients tolerate it very well. If your insurance really refuses to pay, we might try the following:

- Slow-iron or those with less iron element preparations
- Take every other day or one to two times a week
- Eat a small snack with the iron supplement. This will reduce the absorption, but better than nothing.
- Sometimes, the patient might be better to switch to a liquid formulation

What are the intravenous iron formulations?

Every formulation works. The limiting factor is the cost. My clinic uses iron dextran because it is the cheapest.

I usually recommend 1000-1200 mg iv in 1L normal saline infused in four hours.

The first time this product is used, we need a small test dose to make sure there is no reaction.

For those patients with a history of lots of drug reactions, I usually use a premedication like a steroid to help. Do not let your doctor give you intravenous Benadryl which is reported to cause major issues like low blood pressure. People are afraid of infusion reactions. We do a lot of iron infusion because it is very effective, and most patients feel better in a few days.

Other formulations are: ferric carboxymaltose, ferric gluconate, ferumoxytol, and iron sucrose. I have not used any of these products.

What is the potential side effects of intravenous iron infusion?

The most worrisome side effect is an allergic reaction, including potentially life-threatening anaphylaxis. Luckily, it is very rare. We also use a small test dose. If there is no reaction in 15 minutes, then any severe reaction is unlikely.

Do not let your doctor to order a premed like Benadryl, since it can cause many severe reactions such as headache, drowsiness, stomach upset, heart rate changes and low blood pressure. Many doctors confuse the reaction to Benadryl with an allergic reaction to iron infusion.

IV iron may be associated with nonallergic infusion reactions like self-limiting urticaria (hives), palpitations, dizziness, neck and back spasms, and joint pain.

My insurance does not pay for the intravenous iron and I cannot tolerate oral iron. What can I eat more?

As we discussed before, the most important is to find out why you have iron deficiency. If you do not have any other way or resources, then eat more high iron content food. You can try to buy some iron fortified cereal, animal liver, red meat, beans, spinach, seafood, fish and oysters. Chocolate also has good amount of irons.

What was the outcome for your patient?

She is very happy now. She has so much energy and is able to exercise daily. She was able to lose 10 pounds. She cannot believe that a little iron makes so much difference.

Case 4. 55-year-old male was presented with Hashimoto's thyroiditis, fatigue and weight loss.

This is a 55-year-old male who was referred to me for Hashimoto's thyroiditis. He continued to feel badly although his thyroid function was normal. The primary care physician had tried all different thyroid medications, but none worked.

He is taking Synthroid 175 ug daily and his TSH, FT3 and FT4 were normal. He claimed that he had been taking his medication consistently.

He was found to have slightly low iron. He was referred to a gastroenterologist (GI) for further workup and he was found to have colon cancer. He is lucky that we found it early, so he just had surgery and does not need chemo or radiation therapy.

Why do you refer a man to a GI for an iron deficiency workup?

Men do not have menstrual periods. The most common causes for blood loss is the GI tract ulcer or colon cancer. Sometimes diverticulitis or an A-V malformation may also be the cause. For patients on blood thinners, GI blood loss is very common.

Everyone who has unexplained iron deficiency should have a up endoscopy to make sure no ulcer, or colonoscopy to make sure there is no colon cancer or other pathology.

Can I eat more red meat for my iron?

It is true diet iron is a good source for iron. Red meat and liver have the highest levels of iron; However, we do not recommend eating too much red meat because of other health issues.

We always said spinach has a high level of iron, but I saw a report saying that the high level of iron in spinach is due to the misplaced decimal point by a researcher! I don't really know the truth. The bottom line is that the absorption of iron from plant is not very good. The good news is that spinach is very healthy to eat. I really like it. You can eat as much as you want.

Since two thirds of the population is overweight or obese and with abnormal cholesterol it has never been a good idea to recommend eating more red meat or other animal products.

What is the outcome of your patient?

Now that he had surgery and he does not need chemotherapy or radiation. His iron has been replaced and he feels significantly better in terms of energy. He is able to exercise. He still needs to adapt his diet and increase activity to lose more weight.

Case 5. 55-year-old female was suspected of having Hashimoto's thyroiditis with significant fatigue, dry skin, dry hair and dry nails.

This is a 55-year-old female. She had not been feeling well for at least seven or eight years after she had a hysterectomy. She has significant fatigue, a poor sense of well-being, very dry skin, dry hair, hair loss, dry nails and cracked nails. Over the years of Hashimoto's thyroiditis. She has been taking Synthroid 25 ug daily. Her TSH, FT3, and FT4 were all normal. TPO was slightly elevated. She also was on estrogen, progesterone, and testosterone for possible postmenopausal syndrome.

On her first visit, we found her iron and saturation were elevated. Hemochromatosis was suspected, and I referred her to a hematologist for further workup. The gene test was performed. She indeed had homozygous of HFE gene-C282Y mutation.

What is hemochromatosis?

It is caused by absorbing too much iron. The excessive iron can deposit in every cell, tissue and organ and cause damage. It is a hereditary disease. We called it "autosomal recessive". This means you need to have two bad genes to have a severe problem.

Shunzhong Bao, MD

What is the gene responsible for hemochromatosis?

The gene responsible for hemochromatosis is the HFE gene. HFE means high iron (H-high, Fe-iron). The gene product is actually the monitor of our body's iron. If too much, then our body will reduce the absorption. If the monitor is not normal (has mutation), then our body loses the ability to regulate the absorption.

Is there any other gene mutation that can cause hemochromatosis?

HFE is a monitor. Any other gene involved in iron absorption can cause a problem, but much less frequently. Another gene called hepcidin is considered the "master" iron regulatory hormone. Hepcidin determines how much iron can be absorbed.

How common is the hemochromatosis?

Population screening reported that the frequency of heterozygotes of hemochromatosis is approximately ten percent in Caucasian populations in the United States and western Europe, with a frequency of approximately five per 1000 (one in 200 people) for the homozygous state. The percentage is very high. Think about diabetes rate, we have around 10% of the population. Everybody knows somebody who has diabetes.

As you said, hemochromatosis is hereditary. I had the problem when I was born. Why I do not have any problem all these years?

It takes time for iron to accumulate in your body and cause damage. You need 20 g of extra iron to cause major problems. This takes 40 years. Every day, as an adult we dispose around 1 mg of iron by skin shed, sweating and in urine and stool. For a hemochromatosis patient, an average of 2-4 mg is absorbed daily. When at the growing stage of life, you need more iron. So, before age 20, usually even for hemochromatosis patients, there is usually not too much excessive iron accumulation. After age 20, for example, let us say 3 mg are excessively retained. So, for one year, the patient has around 365x3=1 g of iron. To get to 20 grams, you need 20 years. Thus, it will not be until age 40 or 50 that total iron accumulation will reach more than 20 g of iron. On the other hand, women become symptomatic later in life because of the extra iron losses associated with menses, pregnancy, and lactation.

For my patient, she developed symptoms after she reached the postmenopausal stage.

What is the manifestation of hemochromatosis besides fatigue?

Iron can deposit in any cells and cause problems. Most commonly, in the liver, it causes liver dysfunction; in skin, it causes "brown skin"; in the pancreas, it causes diabetes; in the pituitary, it causes hypopituitarism; in gonads, it causes hypogonadism (low T); in joints, it causes arthralgia and osteoarthritis; in the heart, it causes cardiomyopathy.

Does hemochromatosis cause a thyroid problem?

Yes, it can cause a thyroid problem and cause TPO to increase. My patient was referred to me because her TPO was elevated and she was diagnosed with Hashimoto's thyroiditis.

How is hemochromatosis treated?

The treatment was relatively easy. Phlebotomy periodically is the treatment.

What was the outcome of your patient?

After a few months of treatment, she has been completely transformed. She is very happy and grateful. Finally, she was correctly diagnosed and properly treated. Her hair loss has stopped, and her liver function is back to normal. She is gaining back her energy. She told me that she gained her life back.

In her case, her TPO was high, but her problem is not Hashimoto's thyroiditis. Hemochromatosis is very common, and it can cause TPO to increase.

Case 6. 34-year-old female was referred for Hashimoto's thyroiditis with fatigue and memory loss.

This is a 34-year-old female who was referred to me for Hashimoto's thyroiditis. She was diagnosed with Hashimoto's thyroiditis for 10 years and treated with Armour thyroid. Her TSH was normal, FT4 was slightly low and FT3 was normal.

She had significant fatigue, was not feeling well and always felt foggy with poor memory. She has not been sleeping well. She was also diagnosed with anxiety and restless leg syndrome. She was suspected of having Hashimoto's encephalopathy.

Her physical exam was essentially normal.

I repeated her thyroid function and the values were stated as above. I also did other tests like blood counts. She was found to have mild anemia (Hemoglobin was 11.2 g/dl). Her red cell size was increased which is measured by MCV (mean corpuscular volume).The normal value was 88-96. Her value was 105. Her B12 was low at 185 pg/dl. Her folate was normal.

Then we also checked intrinsic factor antibody to be positive. She has pernicious anemia.

She was treated with a B12 monthly injection.

Shunzhong Bao, MD

What is pernicious anemia?

Pernicious anemia is also an autoimmune disease which is caused by destruction of the cells in the stomach which produce intrinsic factor which is required for B12 absorption. All autoimmune diseases can travel together. The rate of pernicious anemia is increased in patients with Hashimoto's thyroiditis.

What are the symptoms of B12 deficiency?

The symptoms can be very nonspecific, such as depression, memory loss, forgetfulness, anxiety irritableness, weakness, fatigue, numbness, or tingling. If very severe, it can cause gait disturbance, and falling, dementia, and psychosis. It can cause restless leg syndrome and sleep disturbance

Is it true that vitamin B12 deficiency also causes heart problem?

Elevated homocysteine levels are thought to promote thrombogenesis, impair endothelial vasomotor function, promote lipid peroxidation, and induce vascular smooth muscle proliferation. Evidence from retrospective, cross-sectional, and prospective studies links elevated homocysteine levels with coronary heart disease and stroke. Vitamin B12, folate, and vitamin B6 are involved in homocysteine metabolism. Supplementing these vitamins helps to reduce homocysteine.

Are pernicious anemia and B12 deficiency the same?

Pernicious anemia is just one reason of the many reasons which can cause vitamin B12 deficiency. This happens to be an autoimmune disease which can travel with Hashimoto's thyroiditis. However, this does not mean pernicious anemia is the most common cause for vitamin B12 deficiency in Hashimoto's thyroiditis patients. Nevertheless, I always check the intrinsic factor if I find vitamin B12 deficiency in Hashimoto's thyroiditis.

What are the other common reasons causing vitamin B12 deficiency?

Vitamin B12 deficiency occurs more often in the following conditions:
- History of gastric surgery (gastrectomy, bariatric surgery)
- Uncontrolled GI conditions (Crohn's disease, celiac disease, pancreatic insufficiency with or without chronic pancreatitis)
- Other autoimmune disease like Hashimoto's thyroiditis
- Medications affecting the B12 absorption: metformin - diabetes medication
- Strict vegan diet
- Breastfeeding
- Some rare intestinal parasites

How do you diagnose vitamin B12 deficiency?

If for any reason, you suspect that you have vitamin B12 deficiency, you can ask your doctor to check the B12 value. It is just a blood test. Be aware, that the blood level of B12 can be variable. I also recommend checking folate levels. The deficiency of folate can occur with B12 deficiency or by itself.

Do I need to check anything else for the diagnosis of vitamin B12 deficiency?

If you do not have some obvious reasons for B12 deficiency, such as a gastrectomy or gastric bypass, I would check the possibility of celiac disease and pernicious anemia. Both these conditions are more often in patients with Hashimoto's thyroiditis.

If you have some GI symptoms, I might check the possibility of H. Pylori infection with a breathing test. It is reported that H. Pylori infection can also cause B12 deficiency.

Some physicians also check methylmalonic acid (MMA) and homocysteine. B12 is needed for MMA to be converted to succinyl-CoA. If there is B12 deficiency, MMA will be accumulated.

Both B12 and folate are required for homocysteine to be converted to methionine. Therefore, either deficiency of B12 or folate can cause homocysteine to increase.

I usually do not check them, since my threshold to treat is very low, the replacement is cheap, and they are water-soluble vitamin and is not easy to overdose.

How do we treat B12 deficiency?

For mild cases, usually I recommend some sublingual vitamin B12 like 5000 u daily. If your cause cannot be corrected, you need a long term supplement.

If you have severe B12 deficiency or have real pernicious anemia, typically vitamin B12 is administered parenterally by intramuscular or deep subcutaneous injection, at a dose of 1000 mcg (1 mg) once per week for four weeks, followed by 1000 mcg once per month.

If sublingual supplement is not effective for mild cases, I give 1 mg once a month intramuscular injection in addition.

Should I buy the active vitamin B12 instead of regular synthetic vitamin B12?

Usually we use the synthetic form-cyanocobalamin, which contains a cyanide (CN) atom introduced during chemical synthesis. It is very effective in treating B12 deficiency.

Methylcobalamin and 5-deoxyadenosylcobalamin are the forms of vitamin B12 that are active in human metabolism. There is no evidence that they are better. As a matter of fact, if you get B12 from a doctor, you can only get cyanocobalamin.

What is the outcome of your patient?

She was treated with a B12 injection for four weeks and then followed by 1 mg muscle injection every month. Her weakness and fatigue improved in the first month and her complaining of brain fog and memory loss significantly improved in a few months. Her symptom of restless syndrome was gone.

Case 7. 25-year-old female presented with significant fatigue, poor memory and irritable bowel

This is a 25-year-old female. She was diagnosed of Hashimoto's hypothyroidism at age 16. For the past nine years, she has never been feeling well. Her thyroid medication has never been stable. Every time she visits her doctor the dose is changed. She has every dose of the thyroid medication at home. She also was put on desiccated thyroid medication like Armour thyroid, but it did not do any better. The problem is that even occasionally her thyroid function was normal, but she continued to not feel well. She always has been tired, wanting to sleep all the time. She depended on a few cups of coffee to get through her day. Her hair and skin were dry, and nails were brittle.

Besides of her thyroid related history, she also reported having "irritable bowel" syndrome, and iron deficiency.

We suspected that she might have celiac disease. We did the blood screening test and it was truly positive and the diagnosis was confirmed by a gastroenterologist.

Why did you suspect this patient might have celiac disease?

Hashimoto's thyroiditis itself can cause the thyroid to be unstable. However, celiac disease is also an autoimmune disease and they tend to travel together. In her case, she seemed to have malabsorption/irregular absorption with the frequently changing dose. Some "irritable bowel syndrome" is caused by celiac disease.

When do you order celiac disease screening?

If you already have Hashimoto's thyroiditis, which is an autoimmune disease, if you also have any one of the following, I will order a celiac disease screening:

- Your dose has to be changed frequently and you have been taking your medication all the time correctly.
- You have any sort of evidence of malabsorption, like iron deficiency, B12 deficiency.
- You have "irritable bowel syndrome".
- You have any of the following skin conditions: dermatitis herpetiformis, alopecia areata, cutaneous vasculitis, urticaria, atopic dermatitis, psoriasis, oral mucosa, chronic ulcerative stomatitis.
- You have type I diabetes.
- You have family history of celiac disease.
- You have recurrent migraine headaches.
- You have idiopathic peripheral neuropathy (like numbness and tingling)
- You have an unknown reason of elevated liver function test.
- You have recurrent fetal loss, reduced fertility.
- You are a mother of low birthweight infants.

How do I prepare for the screening test?

The screening test is just a blood test. You do not need to do anything extra. The only thing you need to know is that if you are on a gluten free diet already, You should not do the test since it might be false negative.

What do you order for the screening test?

We usually order IgA antibody for anti-tissue transglutaminase (IgA TTG), IgA endomysial antibody (IgA EMA). If negative, we will also measure the total IgA to make sure the patient is not IgA deficient.

What is the next step if I have positive results on the screening test?

We will refer to a gastroenterologist if you have a positive screening test or even negative, but we still think the patient has celiac disease.

What is the outcome of your patient?

My patient was confirmed to have celiac disease by a small bowel biopsy, and she started a strict gluten free diet. Now her thyroid function is stabilized, and her iron deficiency is corrected. Amazingly her "irritable bowel syndrome" is cured. She feels like a new person.

Case 8. 58-year-old female presented with Hashimoto's thyroiditis, fatigue, dry mouth, dry skin, day time drowsiness and poor memory

58-year-old female was referred to me for Hashimoto's thyroiditis. She has been on brand name Synthroid 200 ug daily and she has been taking her medication consistently and correctly. Her thyroid function TSH, FT3 and FT4 were all normal. She wanted to increase her dose, but her doctor refused. This is why she was referred to me.

Her major concern was that despite normal thyroid function, she continued to feel very significant fatigue. In further questioning, she revealed that she never had a good sleep. She woke up frequently. Even in the morning, she was feeling tired and sometimes she also had a headache. She could not drive 30 mins without falling asleep. Whenever she sat down she would doze off.

I suspected that she had obstructive sleep apnea. She was convinced to have a sleep study and indeed she had severe sleep apnea and she was started on a CPAP machine.

What is obstructive sleep apnea (OSA)?

During sleep the airway collapses and causes lack of air into your lungs. It causes low oxygen in your body. It disrupts the sleep cycle. Patients wake up, gasping for air. The sleep partner always describes the patient as snoring, restless, or gasping for air after they stop breathing.

Patients always have daytime symptoms of sleepiness, fatigue, or poor concentration, poor memory, sometimes even intractable migraine headaches.

How common is obstructive sleep apnea?

It is very common. It is estimated 20-30% of American males have it; 10-15% of American females have it. The prevalence in patients with Hashimoto's thyroiditis might be even higher.

What are the risk factors?

- Obesity is the number one risk factor. It was reported that OSA was present in 11 percent of men who had normal weight, 21 percent of those who were overweight (BMI 25 to 30 kg/m2), and 63 percent of those who were obese (BMI >30 kg/m2). For adult women, OSA was present in three percent of those who had normal weight, nine percent of those who were overweight, and 22 percent of those who were obese.
- Male gender and age
- Allergy-I did not see a study yet, However, I always treat allergy if suspected before sending for sleep study.
- Hypothyroidism
- Heart failure and other medical conditions
- Using sleep medication (not well studied)

When should I suspect OSA?

Anyone who wakes up not feeling fresh and rested should be evaluated. You might feel significant daytime sleepiness, fatigue, experience poor memory, be irritable and so on.

Other symptoms are waking up with dry mouth, awakening with a sensation of choking, gasping, or smothering. If you sleep with somebody, you might be told that you have episodes of stopping breathing and gasping for air. OSA also has been linked to hypertension, mood disorder, cognitive dysfunction, coronary artery disease, stroke, congestive heart failure, atrial fibrillation, type 2 diabetes mellitus, hypogonadism (low libido and or erectile dysfunction), fibromyalgia, and an array of diseases and conditions.

How OSA is diagnosed?

If you are suspected to have obstructive sleep apnea, usually you will be referred to have a sleep study monitored by a sleep medicine physician. There are two kinds of tests. For most patients, they will have an attended, in-laboratory polysomnography which is considered the **gold-standard** diagnostic test for OSA.

These days, we are trying to cut the cost. If you have a very high risk for OSA, but are relatively healthy, you can have home sleep apnea testing (HSAT).

How OSA is being treated?

Everybody knows the sleep machine (like CPAP) is the treatment for OSA. However, I emphasize these modifiable factors:
- Weight loss, since being overweight is the number one cause for OSA.
- Treating your allergies. There are not too many studies about this. My experience is that treating the allergy is crucial before you start anything else.
- Adjusting or stopping medications which might cause worsening of your OSA.
- Avoiding alcohol

What medications worsen your OSA?

- Benzodiazepine receptor agonists, barbiturates
- Other antiepileptic drugs
- Sedating antidepressants
- Antihistamines
- Opiates

- Antidepressants that cause weight gain (eg, mirtazapine) might be particularly problematic in these patients.
- Some antidepressants may worsen sleep by causing restless legs syndrome or periodic limb movements.

How long should my OSA being treated?

If your cause cannot be corrected, this is a chronic condition and you need to be followed up long term.

What is the outcome of your patient?

She was evaluated by a sleep medicine physician and treated with CPAP. She was able to use the machine and she was able to lose more than 30 lbs after life-style modification. She feels ten years younger and she can do what she wants to do. She says her life has been completely revived.

Case 9. 65-year-old female was referred for Hashimoto's thyroiditis, and significant fatigue

This 65-year-old female actually had a much more complicated medical history than just Hashimoto's thyroiditis. She had six years' history of type II diabetes for which she had been on basal insulin 80 units daily. She also was on metformin 1 g two times a day and Actos 30 mg daily, glimepiride 4 mg two times a day. Her A1c was reasonably under control at 7.2%. She also had hypertension under reasonable control on lisinopril 20 mg daily, and amlodipine 10 mg daily. She had been diagnosed with obstructive sleep apnea (OSA) for five years and was treated with CPAP. She had pain in all her joints. For Hashimoto's thyroiditis, she believed that she had been taking all sorts of supplements. Now she is back to levothyroxine 250 ug po daily.

She has been trying to lose weight all her life. She tried different diets. Currently, she could not do much exercise due to joint pain. At her first visit, she weighed 322 pounds. Her height was 5 feet 2 inches. Her BMI was 58.9.

The reason she was referred was because she was so tired and not able to lose weight and she attributed it to Hashimoto's thyroiditis. Her hypertension and diabetes were reasonably controlled. Her OSA was treated. Everybody thinks this must be a thyroid problem. So, she was referred to make her thyroid better although her thyroid function test was normal.

As I tell my patients, I treat everything. I want to look at my patients as a whole, not just one condition, one disease or one organ. The thyroid is very important and is crucial for cells to work properly. Abnormal thyroid function absolutely causes fatigue and weight problems. However, we cannot just focus on the thyroid just because you have a thyroid problem. The point is that we cannot ignore everything else because you have a thyroid problem.

I was able to convince her to start on a new weight loss journey. I adjusted her diabetes medication. I reduced her insulin dose, stopped Actos. Victoza (GLP-1 agonist) was started and she was able to tolerate it. Jardiance was started. Metformin was continued. She also started a new low carb, low meat and high fiber diet. In 12 months, she was able to lose around 120 lbs and her insulin was stopped. She told me that she never felt so well before. She was able to do so much she couldn't even imagine before. She had a knee replacement and was able to walk more. She was able to keep her weight down.

How do we make the diagnosis of obesity?

The word "obesity" means excessive fat. However, we do not have an easy way to measure your body fat yet.

We all know that obesity is the big problem in modern society. However, not too long ago, obesity could not be diagnosed.

Since the stigma was attached to obesity, some doctors do not want to offend patients and do not mention it to their patients at all.

The easiest way to make the diagnosis is to use the BMI. You can calculate your BMI or use an online calculator.

BMI is calculated as follows:

BMI = body weight (in kg) ÷ height squared, in meters

BMI-based classifications — for Caucasian, Hispanic, and black
individuals (different ethnicities have different classifications):

- Underweight – <18.5 kg/m2
- Normal weight – ≥18.5 to 24.9 kg/m2
- Overweight – ≥25.0 to 29.9 kg/m2
- Obesity – ≥30 kg/m2

    o Class I – 30.0 to 34.9 kg/m2
    o Class II – 35.0 to 39.9 kg/m2
    o **Class III** – **≥40 kg/m2** (also referred to as severe,
       extreme, or massive obesity)

Why is BMI not perfect?

- BMI underestimates the fatness for short people.
- BMI overestimates the fatness for taller people.
- BMI overestimates the fatness for muscular people
- BMI underestimates the fatness for sarcopenia people (less
  muscle).
- BMI overestimates the fatness for people with fluid retention.
- BMI overestimates the fatness for people with "third space
  water collection"-like ascites.
- BMI overestimates the fatness for people who have large
  benign tumors.

I'm guessing there are other reasons why BMI is not perfect. However,
in clinic, we know who is obese and who is not just by looking.

What is the diagnostic criteria of using waist circumferences?

A waist circumference of ≥40 in (102 cm) for white, black, and Hispanic men and ≥35 in (88 cm) for white, black, and Hispanic women is considered elevated and indicative of increased cardiometabolic risk. Other ethnic groups have different criteria.

What evaluation should I receive if I am obese?

I usually screen for weight related complications:

- Diabetes/prediabetes
- Dyslipidemia
- Hypertension
- Fatty liver
- OSA
- Respiratory disease
- Cardiac history
- Osteoarthritis
- Sex related conditions like PCOS, hypogonadism, infertility, urinary stress incontinence, etc
- Digestive conditions (constipation, GERD, etc.)
- Depression

What is your approach to obesity?

Dealing with obesity is not easy and complicated. I am working on a book specific for obesity from my own experience helping my patients lose weight.

I use the following 7-D's as a guide:

1. Desire-I assess patient's desire to lose weight. Not everyone wants to lose weight. Certainly, I also help patients to increase their desire to lose weight.
2. Decision. It is crucial for you to make the decision to lose weight, to start to change your lifestyle. I am here to facilitate the process and provide guidance.
3. Determination. You always will have bumps on the road. Determination is crucial. Otherwise, you will go back to square one.
4. Discipline. Losing weight is like doing anything else. You need discipline. No discipline, you will never succeed.
5. Diet and exercise. We call it lifestyle change. However, the basics are your diet and exercise.
6. Drugs. I always look into the drugs you are taking. Many drugs cause weight gain. Other drugs might help you lose weight.
7. Disease. I also look for possible diseases or conditions which might cause weight gain.

Case 10. 21-year-old college student presented with fatigue, depressed mood, insomnia, anxiety, poor memory and lack of concentration.

21-year-old female was referred for Hashimoto's thyroiditis with fatigue, depressed mood, insomnia, anxiety, poor memory and lack of concentration.

She was diagnosed with Hashimoto's thyroiditis last year. She is taking Synthroid 50 ug daily. Her thyroid function was repeated to be within normal limits. However, she continues to have significant fatigue, depressed mood, insomnia, anxiety, poor memory and lack of concentration. She missed some school due to above symptoms. She is not in a relationship. She denied any thoughts of hurting herself or other people.

I suggested that she might be depressed. I suggested that I could refer her for psychotherapy or to a psychiatrist. However, she wanted me to try SSRI (depression medication). I talked to her mom and let her pay attention to her response to the medication. After three months treatment, she reported to be back to normal. She feels so much better, not depressed anymore. She is able to participate in school activities and concentrate on her classes. She has not missed another school day since she started treatment. During this period, her thyroid medication has not been changed.

What is depression?

Depression is a real condition. Depression is an emotional disorder. Depression affects the quality of life of yourself and other people surrounding you. There is an array of symptoms to meet the diagnosis, but you need to have a depressed mood or loss of interest in pleasure.

How common is depression?

In the United States, the National Comorbidity Survey Replication found an annual prevalence rate for major depressive disorder (MDD) of 6.7 percent and a lifetime prevalence rate of 16.5 percent. Other conditions and disease status affect the rate of depression. Among patients with chronic medical illness, the annual prevalence rate is approximately 25 percent. Depression is associated with untreated hypothyroidism. I am not certain about the exact rate.

How is depression diagnosed?

Untreated or not well managed hypothyroidism has been linked to depression. Therefore, I always pay attention and ask for symptoms of depression.

A lot of times, patients present with fatigue, insomnia or sleeping too much, weight gain, weight loss, poor memory, fibromyalgia, or thyroid disorders.

The diagnostic criteria are at least 5 of the following symptoms:
- Depressed mood or loss of interest or pleasure in most or all activities (you need to have this)
- Insomnia or hypersomnia (cannot sleep or sleep too much)
- Gain weight or weight loss
- Anxiety, agitation or slowing down emotion and physical movement

99

- Fatigue/low energy
- Poor concentration/poor job performance/poor school work
- Thoughts of worthlessness or guilt
- Recurrent thoughts about death or suicide

How is depression treated?

Depression is not my specialty; however, many endocrine diseases are linked to depression and I try my best to help my patients. Not everyone has access to a psychiatrist.

First, I treat the conditions in which I excel. Every single one of the endocrine conditions affects depression. Obesity, uncontrolled diabetes and its comorbidities, uncontrolled hypothyroidism, hypogonadism, etc., play a major role in depression. Depression can affect endocrine condition management. Therefore, I always try my best to break this vicious cycle.

Second, I try my way of "psychotherapy". A specialist might tell you that mood is different from emotions. I think the connection of emotions are your mood. Therefore, depression is an emotional disorder. I try to teach my patients to take ownership of their emotions, just like standing up or sitting down. You can choose how you feel. Certainly, it is not easy, but you can actively make yourself feel that way.

Third, I let my patients try depression medication. Depression medication has changed the landscape of depression management. It is okay to try.

Case 11. 46-year-old female was referred for Hashimoto's thyroiditis and dry mouth

This 46-year-old female was diagnosed with Hashimoto's thyroiditis for over ten years. She has been on Synthroid 150 ug daily for some time. Her dose was changed periodically but not too drastically. Now her major concern is that she has this dry mouth and also dry skin. She attributed these symptoms to her Hashimoto's thyroiditis.

However, in questioning, I determined she also has severe seasonal allergy and is taking a few allergy medications including Benadryl. She also has anxiety. Her primary care physician put her on promethazine for anxiety.

I confirmed that her thyroid function was acceptable, and I suggested that her dry mouth and dry skin might be related to her medications like promethazine and Benadryl. She was willing to try taking less promethazine. She continued her Benadryl at night for sleep and allergy. She reported that her dry mouth was significantly better. Now that she understands her medication was the reason for her dry mouth. She is not so worried about her thyroid. She feels much at ease and just deals with the dry mouth with another over-the-counter remedy.

What are the medications which can cause dry mouth?

Atropine and scopolamine:

They are usually used for abdominal pain and spasms and are known to reduce the secretions of many glands including the salivary glands.

Antidepressants:

Antidepressants are drugs used for the treatment of major depressive disorders. They are also used for many other conditions like anxiety disorder, eating disorders, chronic pain, dysthymia, fibromyalgia, obsessive compulsive disorders (OCD), neuropathic pain, postmenopausal syndrome, etc. I have many patients who are being treated for these conditions.

The most common antidepressants that list dry mouth as a side effect are tricyclic antidepressants (Amitriptyline, Doxepin, Nortriptyline, Amoxapine, etc.), selective serotonin reuptake inhibitors (Celexa, Lexapro, Prozac, Paxil, Zoloft, etc.), and lithium (Lithobid, etc.), bupropions (Wellbutrin, Aplenzin, Budeprion SR, Buproban, Forfivo XL, Wellbutrin, Wellbutrin SR, Wellbutrin XL, Zyban, Zyban Advantage Pack, Budeprion XL}

Hypertension Medications:

Many alpha blockers, and beta blockers can cause dry mouth. Some examples are terazosin (Hytrin), prazosin (Minipress), clonidine (Catapres, Kapvay, Nexiclon XR), atenolol (Tenormin), and propranolol (Inderal).

Any water-pills can cause dry mouth and dehydration.

Phenothiazines:

Phenothiazines are commonly used to treat severe nausea, vomiting, and treating serious mental and emotional disorders (including schizophrenia).

The most common drug on my patients' medication list is promethazine (Phenergan).

Allergy medications:

Many people are taking some sort of allergy medications:

Examples of antihistamines that may cause dry mouth include Allegra, Benadryl, Dimetane, Claritin, Alavert, and Zyrtec.

Proton pump inhibitor (Acid reflux medications):

Proton pump inhibitors (PPI) are used to treat acid reflux, ulcers, and H. Pylori infections.

Examples of proton pump inhibitors that may cause dry mouth include esomeprazole, lansoprazole, omeprazole, rabeprazole, Nexium, Prevacid, Prilosec, and Aciphex.

Opioids:

Many patients have chronic pain and opioids are used.

Examples of opioids that may cause dry mouth include codeine, fentanyl, Actiq, Fentora, hydrocodone, Lorcet, Vicodin, hydromorphone, Dilaudid, Demerol, methadone, morphine, Avinza, oxycodone, OxyContin, Percocet, and Roxicodone.

Cannabinoids:

More and more people are using marijuana for various reasons. Marijuana is a cannabinoid. It can cause dry mouth.

Cytotoxic drugs

Hashimoto's thyroiditis is an autoimmune disease, and autoimmune diseases tend to travel together. Many of my patients also have conditions like systemic lupus erythematosus, dermatomyositis, rheumatoid arthritis, Wegener's granulomatosis, and vasculitis. They are being treated with one of these medications: azathioprine, Imuran, cyclophosphamide, Cytoxan, methotrexate, Rheumatrex, and Trexall.

Retinoids:

Retinoids are commonly used for acne and psoriasis. Younger patients with Hashimoto's thyroiditis tend to have more acne. Psoriasis is also increased in the population of patients with Hashimoto's thyroiditis. Examples of retinoids that may cause dry mouth include acitretin, Soriatane, tretinoin, and isotretinoin.

AIDS medications:

Protease inhibitors (PIs) are antiretroviral medicines that are most commonly used to prevent the HIV and hepatitis C viruses from multiplying in the body

Didanosine is most commonly used along with other medications to treat human immunodeficiency virus (HIV) infection by decreasing the amount of HIV in the blood.

Ephedrine /Phentermine:

Ephedra or ephedrine are banned in America, but you still can get them from somewhere.

Phentermine is the most popular weight loss medication.

Benzodiazepines:

For some reasons, patients with Hashimoto's thyroiditis have an increased rate of anxiety. Benzodiazepines are most commonly used to treat panic disorders (anxiety), and also epilepsy or to help control certain manic symptoms in bipolar disorder such as mania, insomnia, and seizures. Some patients also take them for sleep.

There are many other medications which might cause dry skin and dry mouth. If you have these symptoms, I recommend having your doctors look into your medications.

What other conditions associated with Hashimoto's thyroiditis might be causing dry mouth?

Many conditions can cause dry mouth. These are the conditions I usually think of: Sjogren's disease, diabetes mellitus, diabetes insipidus, heart failure, allergies, history of radioactive iodine treatment, thyroid dysfunction (either overactive or underactive), post stroke, asthma (any condition causing you to breathe fast), OSA with people with morning dryness, anxiety, depression, etc.

What can we do with dry mouth?

If possible you and your doctor should identify the cause and treat the cause. If you think medication might be the culprit, if possible change the medication or reduce the dose, Certainly, you need to work with your doctor.

What can we do if the cause cannot be corrected or identified?

- Keep yourself well hydrated if your doctor does not put a water restriction on you.
- Keep your environment with good humidity. Use a humidifier especially in the winter.
- Try your best to breathe with your nose instead of your mouth. Keep your mouth closed. Listen more, talk less.

- Try your best not to drink coffee, alcohol, smoke cigarettes or marijuana.
- Try your best not to drink sugary drinks.
- Try your best not to drink acidic drinks (soda, coffee, tea, fruit juice, most sports drinks, etc)
- Try some non-sugary lozenges/chewing gums
- Try some xylitol containing gum or lozenges.
- Try some citrus flavored gum or lozenges.
- Try some artificial saliva.

I have tried all of the above, none of them can relieve my dry mouth. Is there anything else I can try?

Under care of your doctor, you can try pilocarpine 5 mg by mouth, up to four times daily, or cevimeline 30 mg by mouth, up to three times daily taken about a half-hour before meals. These are medications and have side effects you need to discuss with your doctor.

What else should I pay attention to if I have dry mouth?

You need to see your dentist often to make sure you're not developing cavities or some fungus infection.

Case 12. 56-year-old female with Hashimoto's thyroiditis and diabetes gained ten pounds in ten days.

I have seen Marva for 5 years for her diabetes and Hashimoto's thyroiditis. For her Hashimoto's thyroiditis, she has been taking levothyroxine 200 ug daily. Her previous thyroid function was fluctuating, but acceptable. I have not changed her dose for one year. For her diabetes, she is taking metformin, Trulicity and a low dose of Lantus at night.

When Marva came to follow up with me, the first question she had was "Can stress affect my thyroid?". I asked what had happened. She told me that she gained ten pounds in ten days. This might be caused by her thyroid. Recently she had lots of stress. So here is the story.

During spring break, her daughter Olivia brought two lovely granddaughters four and six years old to spend time with her. Marva certainly was very happy and anticipated their visit a lot. She bought many "treats" for her granddaughters, including but not limited to cookies and ice cream.

After they arrived, my patient Marva could not wait to hug them and treat them with cookies and ice cream. However, when her daughter saw her mom treating them with cookies and ice cream, she yelled at Marva, "Mom, now if you feed them with this junk food now, then later they will become as fat as you are and develop diabetes, and then you will be happy." Marva was so shocked that she did not have anything to say. The only emotions she had were feeling sad, distrusted, disrespected, and misunderstood by her own daughter. She was frozen, but sadness mixed with madness was not gone. After lunch, they drove to visit Crystal Bridges Museum, At the parking lot, Marva just could not stop her tears pouring down. She thought that she was so excited to have them over and cleaned the house getting beds ready for them, getting food for them and now being called fat by her own daughter. She has been struggling with her own weight and diabetes for a long time. She thought that her daughter was not being supportive, but instead blamed her. There was no way she could stop her tears, so she told her daughter and two lovely granddaughters to go ahead and see the exhibits, that she preferred to sit in the car for a while. After Olivia heard this, she became hostile and drove back home, picked up their stuff and left for their own home in Georgia. It was afternoon already and it takes more than 12 hours to drive to their home. She also has two children four and six years old in the car. Then Marva really regretted what had happened, was self-critical, and apolitical. Unfortunately, her daughter did not respond to Marva's text message or phone calls and she did not know if they made home safely.

She said her stress was up to the roof and this might be affecting her thyroid function. She gained ten pounds in past ten days.

Do stress/emotions affect thyroid function?

The answer is absolutely. Stress can affect your hypothalamus function and pituitary function. The pituitary is the master gland which controls your thyroid gland. Stress might also affect other hormones like cortisol. Cortisol can also inhibit the conversion of T4 to T3. T3 is the active hormone. Therefore, it is true that stress and emotions can affect your thyroid function.

Does thyroid affect your emotions?

The answer again is absolutely. One of the prominent symptoms of overactive thyroid is emotional labile, and irritability. One of the prominent symptoms of the underactive thyroid is depression.

Is Marva's ten-pound weight gain due to her Hashimoto's thyroid acting up?

No, absolutely not. She had lots of emotional stress and everybody is a stress eater. Marva is certainly a stress eater. She finished all the treats for her granddaughters. She bought more treats. Nobody cares about her or respects her. The only thing she can do is to eat. However, she is still a mother and grandmother. She has been worried, regretful, and full of self-pity.

Part of her weight is water. When she is overeating, she is also eating a lot of salt which cause water retention.

How can we take control of our emotion?

We tend to blame other people for making us unhappy. We always tend to give other people the power. However, often times if you practice you are able to take the control back. Here are a few simple steps:

- Always tell yourself, your emotions belong to you. You should be able to control them.
- Try to always give positive emotions to your surroundings.
- Try your best to respond to negative emotion with positive emotion.

What do you mean "emotions belong to you"?

Emotion is what you feel and how you feel. It is your brain activity. It is not other peoples' brain activity. However, it is easy to say but hard to do. Our brain is not built to control and initiate itself. Our brain is always trying to react to our surroundings. When we meet a positive emotion, we tend to respond with positive emotions; when we meet negative emotions, we tend to respond with negative emotions. Our instinct emotion is like a magnetic field. Our instinct is to try to line up with the environment. However, you can choose your emotion if you practice.

Why is it important to put yourself as the source of positive emotion?

As we know, people tend to align with their surroundings. If you can be a source of positive emotion, other people will respond with positive emotion since this is their nature. Someone posted a video on the web. They wanted to see how people would respond to a laugh. One person for no reason laughed in the subway, and then another person began to laugh and in no time, everybody began to laugh. At the end, people asked each other why they laughed. Nobody knew, but they all felt good!

You can use your positive emotions to affect your surroundings.

How can I respond to negative emotions?

If you are in a negative emotion surrounding, you will tend to get aligned with these negative emotions. Here is what you can do:

- Leave the negative emotions surroundings. This is what people say-cool yourself down.
- Respond with fewer negative emotions.

- Respond with positive emotions.

What is your specific advice for your patient Marva if you are in a similar situation?

The best response is to respond with positive emotion to change the environment. This is not easy. You need very dedicated commitment and practice.

- **Leave the negative emotions surroundings.**

Marva had a few opportunities to take control of the situation. She could have said, "I need to go to bathroom" and try to collect myself, or "I need to find something in the closet." She could think about what her goal was. Her goal was to try to make her daughter and granddaughters happy. And they will be here only for three to four days. The time is precious, and she does not want to miss it. Afterwards, she could have come out and put away those cookies and ice cream and try not to think about it. The main thing was they were here.

- **Respond with less negative emotions.**

Marva could have responded to her daughter's negative emotion with less negative emotions. She does not have to be happy. She could just remove those cookies and ice cream and apologize to the kids. Never try to explain or argue, because most of the time, the explanation and argument will not work.

- **Respond with positive emotions.**

This is the most difficult and needs practice. Marva could put on a smiley face and praise her daughter and granddaughters for learning from mistakes of granny and adopt a healthy diet starting early to prevent obesity and diabetes.

Certainly, Marva could have enjoyed the art in the Crystal Bridges Museum and she might have three to four more days with her family. Certainly, she would have the chance to talk to her daughter about the yelling. Marva would have the chance to let Olivia know that for her own benefit, her two youngsters might be learning how to treat their mom. When they grow up they might treat Oliva the same way Olivia treated Marva. Marva might have the opportunity to learn more about her daughter's life. Later on, Marva found out that her daughter Olivia also had been struggling with her and very frustrated not able to lose weight, and recently was told by her doctor that she has prediabetes. She has been worried about her own future diabetes. Lots time, people release their negative emotions because they have something going on in their own lives. It might not be direct to you. You are just the "cat" happened to be there and being kicked.

Life is complicated. I want you to enjoy your life.

Case 13. 58-year-old male with Hashimoto's thyroiditis developed fatigue, exercise intolerance, and simply was not feeling well.

This is a 58-year-old small business owner. He had been working all his life and is quite successfully. He was diagnosed with Hashimoto's hypothyroidism 20 years ago and had been taking Synthroid 200 ug for a long time. He came to me because he had all the symptoms of untreated Hashimoto's hypothyroidism like fatigue and generally not feeling well. He was also gaining weight, 12 pounds in the last year. My clinic is on a small hill and he found himself short of breath by just walking from the bottom of the hill to the clinic. He also had to catch his breath for just three flights of stairs. He denied having chest pain. He also complained of erectile dysfunction and generally low libido. He had obstructive sleep apnea, and already treated with a CPAP machine and feels somewhat better, but just didn't feel well.

In his family history, his father had a heart attack at age 65 and his uncle had a heart attack at age 64.

I did a physical exam. He was well built and apparently obese. His BMI (body mass index) was 38. His blood pressure was slightly elevated but acceptable. Otherwise his physical exam was normal. I checked his basic labs. His blood count (CBC) were normal. His liver enzymes were slightly elevated for which I suspected to be caused by a fatty liver. His blood sugar was 136 with HbA1c of 6.8 for which he met the diagnosis of diabetes.

His lipid profile was not good. His total cholesterol was 280, triglycerides 350, HDL (good cholesterol) 30, and LDL 220. He used statins before, but he was not able to tolerate them due to severe muscle pain.

Why is fatigue so complicated?

Tiredness is one of the most complicated clinical conditions to manage. As we can see from my previous example cases, every organ dysfunction or mental dysfunction can cause fatigue, and it can be a normal response to physiological changes. For example; if you are stressed, you feel tired; if you work too much, play too much, you feel tired; if do not sleep well, you feel tired; if you eat too much, you feel tired; if you have a nutritional deficiency, you feel tired; etc. The list is endless. It can be debilitating, not only affecting personal work performance, but also family life and social relationships.

What is the main reason for this businessman to be so tired?

There are some obvious reasons to cause his fatigue such as: obesity, a fatty liver, and a newly diagnosed but untreated diabetes. However, due to his multiple cardiovascular risk factors and his family history of cardiovascular disease, I recommended him to have a stress test. The stress test was abnormal, and the cardiologist proceeded with a cardiac catheterization. He was found to have severe left anterior descending coronary artery disease (LAD). Two stents were put in. He was also started on medications like Plavix, aspirin, and lisinopril. We were also able to start a new kind of cholesterol medication - PCSK9 inhibitor for him. His bad cholesterol-LDL dropped from 220 to 60. He immediately felt better after the stents. The cardiac lesion in the coronary artery was like a ticking time bomb, and you didn't know when it would blow. The "bomb "was defused and also motivated him to exercise and make himself fit and reduce the risks for future "bomb" formations in his coronary artery system.

What is coronary heart disease(CHD)?

The coronary artery is a set of arteries which support your heart muscle. Your heart depends on them to supply oxygen and nutrition. The coronary artery disease we were talking about is caused by an atherosclerosis process. It takes time to develop, but sometimes the blockage can occur suddenly. This is what we call a heart attack.

What are the modifiable cardiac risk factors?

Certainly, the most prominent risk factor is age. We cannot change chronological age, but there are a number of things you can do to change the vascular age. Family history is also very significant, but we can change lots of habits in your family. Here is a list of major risk factors about which you can do something:

- High cholesterol level
- Smoking
- Uncontrolled Diabetes
- Uncontrolled hypertension
- Obesity (especially abdominal obesity)
- Excessive alcohol
- Stress/unstable emotions
- Inactivity
- Lack of consumption of fresh vegetables and fruit

I am young. Can I have coronary heart disease?

We know that coronary heart disease develops slowly and gradually. In a report of autopsies performed in 1994, the prevalence of significant anatomic CHD in subjects aged 20 to 59 years of age, 32 percent were in men and 16 percent in women. All of these people died of other causes. They did not know that they had coronary heart disease. Diseased plaque is also found in teenage coronary artery.

How do I know if I have clinically significant CHD?

If you have some typical symptoms of CHD like chest pain on exertion, you certainly need to make sure you get checked. Usually you will have a stress test. Some primary care doctors do it, but most likely you need to see a cardiologist for the stress test.

If you do not have typical symptoms or signs, or just feeling tired then we need to look at your risk factors. If you are a man over 40 years of age, and you have two other risk factors, we will refer you to have a stress test. Sometime we will also calculate your risk but this is not really a determinant.

If the results of your stress test are suspicious or positive, you most likely will have a cardiac catheterization. This is the gold standard test for the diagnosis of coronary artery disease.

I do not want to have a stress test. Is there some other test?

You can have a heart calcium score which is a low dose CT scan to look at the calcium buildup in the diseased plaque in the coronary artery.

Your score should be zero. The following is the risk meaning for the calcium score:

0	No plaque is present. You have less than a 5% chance of having heart disease.
1 - 10	A small amount of plaque is present. You have less than a 10% chance of having heart disease. Your risk of a heart attack is low.
11 - 100	Plaque is present. You have mild heart disease. Your chance of having a heart attack is moderate.
101 - 400	A moderate amount of plaque is present. You have heart disease, and plaque may be blocking an artery. Your chance of having a heart attack is moderate to high.
>400	A large amount of plaque is present. You have more than a 90% chance that plaque is blocking one of your arteries. Your chance of having a heart attack is high.

At the end of the day, your cardiologist might still want you to have a stress test depending on your score.

I do not want to have a coronary catheterization. Can I have other tests?

Your cardiologist might recommend a coronary CT scan or an MRA. These tests can help doctors see your coronary artery structure and help decide the next step should be for management and sometimes your cardiologist might decide that you need further action. The regular coronary catheterization is the most common next step. It is invasive, but it can yield more information about your heart like the condition of your heart valve, pressure, ejection fraction, get a blood sample or sample from plaque for further studying. It also will indicate if treatment with stents will be necessary.

What can I do to reduce my risk?

You can do a lot to reduce your risk. Be aware of your risk factors, and work on each one. They are cumulative. The more risk factors you can tackle, the less chance you will have a cardiovascular event.

1. Be aware of your cholesterol levels. Cholesterol, especially LDL, has the most impact on CHD. Your doctor might consider statins or other lipid lowering medications for you.
2. Quit smoking-smoking is the number two modifiable risk factor.
3. Control your blood pressure and/or diabetes.
4. Be active - I recommend exercise every day of the week.
5. Eat more fresh vegetables and moderate amount of fruits. Stay away from high cholesterol and high carb diets, especially fried food or food loaded with trans-fat and refined sugar. I recommend a low carb, low meat, and low-calorie diet. More vegetables are the key not more fruits.
6. You might want to lose weight if you are overweight or obese.

7. If you have other high-risk diseases like rheumatoid arthritis, chronic renal disease (stage III or IV), then you need to take care of them.

Shunzhong Bao, MD

Chapter 6. Hashimoto's Thyroiditis Diet

Does what you eat and what you drink affect your thyroid function?

The answer is a big YES. All steps of thyroid function, (hormone formation, releasing, transportation, conversion, response of cells, inactivation) can be affected by what you eat and what you drink.

I have Hashimoto's hypothyroidism, and take thyroid hormone. Do I need to eat more food that contains more iodine?

Everybody knows iodine is important to thyroid.

If you have Hashimoto's hypothyroidism and have been treated with synthetic thyroid hormone or "nature thyroid hormone", you do not need to eat more iodine rich food. The reason is that you already take the end product of iodine which is the thyroid hormone. Therefore, you really do not need to take extra iodine rich food. We do not think our body else needs iodine to function except for the thyroid. However, the food with high iodine is generally considered healthy. You can eat, and you do not need shy away from them.

Shunzhong Bao, MD

I have Hashimoto's hypothyroidism, and take thyroid hormone. What will happen if I eat a lot of iodine rich food?

Well, that is really a good question. Hashimoto's thyroiditis is not a homogenous disease. In other words, not all Hashimoto's thyroiditis is the same.

First, some patients have two processes going on all the time, but just one dominates. For example, I have quite a few patients, that have been treated with thyroid hormone replacement even as long as 40 years and then suddenly developed an overactive thyroid. It turned out that their stimulating antibodies were also positive. If these people eat excessive iodine rich food, their thyroid might switch to being overactive.

Second, for most patients, the process of Hashimoto's thyroiditis "chews up" your thyroid gland, therefore your thyroid gland becomes smaller and smaller. Eventually only a scar is left in the thyroid bed. As you can see, we have different stages of Hashimoto's thyroiditis, early stage, mid stage, or end stage, or anywhere in between. If your Hashimoto's thyroiditis is at an early stage and you eat too much iodine rich food (see chapter 1), you might get into trouble. If your Hashimoto's thyroiditis is toward the end stage, you will not have any problem at all, because there is no thyroid gland to respond to your high iodine intake.

How much iodine rich food is too much?

I don't think anybody can really tell you. You can do an experiment by yourself. You can eat a certain amount for a few days and go to your doctor to have your 24 hours urine iodine checked. If your 24 hours is above the normal range, then it is too much.

122

My suggestion is do not think about it. If you have one night out enjoying your Sushi or eating kelp or some seaweed, you are okay.

Should I avoid iodine rich food?

No, you do not have to. Since at times, some patients really do not know the stage of their Hashimoto's thyroiditis. I recommend keeping their iodine intake adequate. See Chapter 1 for normal values.

Do I need a gluten free diet?

Gluten free diet is for celiac disease. Both Hashimoto's thyroiditis and celiac disease are autoimmune diseases. Autoimmune diseases tend to travel together. People with Hashimoto's thyroiditis have increased risk for celiac disease, and people with celiac disease have increased risk for Hashimoto's thyroiditis.

Celiac disease is one of the reasons which can cause unstable thyroid function if you are on thyroid hormone supplement. I recommend having a celiac disease screening if you have been taking your medication consistently and faithfully. If your screening is negative, you have two options. You can go to see a gastroenterologist who can do a biopsy, or you can try a period of gluten free diet to see if you can get your thyroid stable or get rid those symptoms which might be associated with celiac disease. See Chapter 5-case 7.

Is it true that patients with Hashimoto's thyroiditis should not eat cruciferous vegetables?

The cruciferous vegetables (brussels sprouts, cabbage, cauliflower, kale, turnips, and bok choy, etc.) were found to have a natural occurring chemical which affects the thyroid gland to take iodine into the cells. However, this only has major effects in the iodine deficiency area. In other words, if you have iodine deficiency and then you eat a lot of cruciferous vegetables, then you might have a thyroid problem.

If you have Hashimoto's thyroiditis, and you are being supplemented with synthetic or "nature thyroid hormone", you do not need to worry about it. You do not need extra iodine since you do not need your thyroid to synthesize thyroid hormone. You are taking them.

If you have adequate iodine intake, you do not need to worry about it.

If your thyroid is normal and you have no iodine deficiency, you do not need to worry about it.

However, if you have Hashimoto's thyroiditis but are not on thyroid hormone replacement therapy, and you are living in an iodine deficiency area (in USA, if you are using iodine fortified salt, you do not have iodine deficiency), then you might want to cook your cruciferous vegetables and limit to five servings a day. It is believed that cooking destroys some iodine-inhibiting naturally occurring chemicals.

Remember, cruciferous vegetables are good for you. Do not stay away from them. They have loads of antioxidants, and you can find more research to link consuming cruciferous vegetables with better health, such as less cardiovascular disease and cancer.

Is it true that Hashimoto's thyroiditis patients should not eat soy or soy products?

Soy is very popular in the Asian diet. Soy is also found to have a naturally occurring chemical which affects iodine uptake into thyroid cells.

Soy also has a naturally occurring chemical to increase the female hormone estrogen. As we know, estrogen is indicated in thyroid disease (females have a much higher rate of Hashimoto's thyroiditis).

Female hormones also increase the thyroid hormone binding protein. Therefore, the thyroid needs to produce more hormones to match the body's need.

However, here are the caveats for you:

1. If you have Hashimoto's thyroiditis, and you are taking synthetic or "nature thyroid hormone", do not worry about it. You are depending on the thyroid supplement. Your thyroid does not need iodine and your dose can always be adjusted. Therefore, you do not need to worry about it.
2. If you have a normal thyroid and you have adequate iodine uptake, you do not need to worry about it.
3. If you have very early stage of Hashimoto's thyroiditis, and you are not on thyroid hormone replacement, you might want to limit to five servings a week.
4. Soy and soy products are much healthier compared to other animal-based protein sources.

Should patients with Hashimoto's thyroiditis consume less fatty food and fried food?

In animal studies, researchers found the rats fed with high fat food have more thyroid dysfunction. Humans might not be so different.

Both high fat and fried food also have been found to affect thyroid medication absorption.

125

Everybody is recommended to consume less high fat or fried food anyway. I think I do not need too much explanation.

Should patients with Hashimoto's thyroiditis stay away from high sugar/high carb diet?

You should. Here are a few reasons I can think of:

1. As we know, the thyroid is very important in regulating metabolism. Your metabolism might be low to start with. If you consume too many carbs or sugar, it might be very easy to gain weight.
2. If you have Hashimoto's thyroiditis, but are not on thyroid medication yet, your thyroid may not be able to catch up to help your body to consume those sugars and carbs.
3. If you have Hashimoto's thyroiditis and you are taking a fixed dose of thyroid hormone replacement, your body can not actively regulate based on your body's need.
4. People with Hashimoto's thyroiditis have a higher risk to developing type I diabetes. My son reported that adult onset type I diabetes is even higher than child onset type I diabetes. He also reported that patients with type I diabetes have much a higher risk for Hashimoto's thyroiditis and other autoimmune diseases.

Should patients with Hashimoto's thyroiditis stay away from plastic wrapped food?

Some chemicals from plastic might affect thyroid function. They are mostly processed food and not healthy anyway.

Can I drink alcohol?

High dose consumption of alcohol significantly affects thyroid function. An occassional single drink might be okay.

It seems nothing is good for thyroid. What can I eat?

- I recommend low carb, low meat to everybody including patients with Hashimoto's thyroiditis.
- I recommend against too much fruit intake because they have too much sugar/carbs.
- I do recommend to consume berries like blackberries, blueberries etc.
- Vegetables, even cruciferous vegetables are okay for you. Just make sure you check your thyroid function periodically and do not forget to take your thyroid medication.
- If you do not have celiac disease, there is no reason for you to go gluten free. I do recommend you consume whole wheat.
- If you have celiac disease, or you suspect it, you want to do the gluten free. There is a whole gluten free diet list.
- Use healthy ways to cook like boiling, or steaming instead of frying, and grilling.

If I stay away from all the "thyroid bad food" and only eat those healthy foods, can I reverse my Hashimoto's thyroiditis?

I know Dr. Google tells you lots of magic, but the truth is that Hashimoto's thyroiditis is an autoimmune disease and it is much more than eating correctly. Further more, when your thyroid function is low, this means your thyroid already has significant damage. It is very important for you to take your thyroid hormone supplement faithfully.

www.ingramcontent.com/pod-product-compliance
Lightning Source LLC
Chambersburg PA
CBHW060608200326
41521CB00007B/695